MILADY'S AESTHETICIAN SERIES

Ensuring an Optimal Outcome in Skin Care

MILADY'S AESTHETICIAN SERIES

Ensuring an Optimal Outcome in Skin Care

PAMELA HILL, R.N.

THOMSON

™

DELMAR LEARNING Australia Canada Mexico Singapore Spain United Kingdom United States

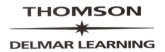

THOMSON

DELMAR LEARNING

Milady's Aesthetician Series: "Ensuring an Optimal Outcome in Skin Care"
Pamela Hill

President, Milady:
Dawn Gerrain

Director of Editorial:
Sherry Gomoll

Acquisitions Editor:
Brad Hanson

Developmental Editor:
Jennifer Radalin

Editorial Assistant:
Jessica Burns

Director of Production:
Wendy A. Troeger

Production Editor:
Nina Tucciarelli

Composition:
Cadmus Professional
  Communications

Director of Marketing:
Wendy Mapstone

Channel Manager:
Sandra Bruce

Cover and Text Design:
Essence of 7

Library of Congress Cataloging-in-Publication Data

Hill, Pamela, RN.
  Ensuring an optimal outcome in skin care / Pamela Hill.
    p. ; cm. –(Milady's aesthetician series)
  Includes bibliographical references and index.
  ISBN 1-4018-8178-5 (pbk.)
  1. Dermatologic nursing. 2. Skin–Care and hygiene. 3. Beauty culture. [DNLM: 1. Dermatologic nursing. 2. Skin–Care and hygiene. 3. Beauty culture. 4. Nurse-Patient Relations. WY 154.5 H6475e 2006] I. Title.
RL125.H55 2006
616.5'0231–dc22

2005015671

NOTICE TO THE READER

Contents

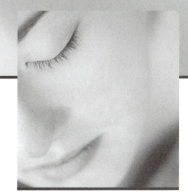

CHAPTER 3

CHAPTER 4

Preface

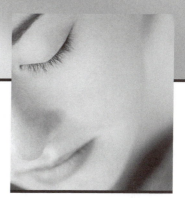

A skilled and knowledgeable clinician can give an excellent treatment, provide an unusually good result, and still have an unhappy patient. Why? So much more is involved in providing treatment than just the process that happens in the clinic. Until now, the clinical aesthetician and cosmetic nurse has had little valuable information about the concepts of medical spa treatment plans, the importance of patient education, and the relationship that follows. As the leader of a network of medical skin-care clinics, I have heard clinicians beg for more information to expand their knowledge base and create a successful paradigm for patient care and communication. For the last 14 years, I have spent my days managing medical spas. Part of my job as the president and chief executive officer was the development and oversight of the training programs for our facilities. Needless to say, I have met and trained many clinicians. What I have noticed is that my first-rate, curious clinicians (aestheticians and nurses) can never get enough information. They are always looking for more information, improved technology to provide advanced results, a new book, and more and more! Although these questions are obvious signs of a good clinician, they are wrought with peril because unbiased information is not always available.

This book is intended for students who are studying to become first-rate clinicians, as well as the clinicians who thirst for more information, expanding on what they already know. That said, this text is written to expand on the basic knowledge of aesthetician training and take it from a conceptual level to the practical level.

I have researched and written this book so that I could satisfy that hunger that makes a great aesthetician and cosmetic nurse. Understanding yourself and the interactions of a team, as well as the personalities and motivations of a patient, is important in the final analysis of outcome. Medical spa treatments and advanced therapies have developed into a multibillion dollar business, but the competition is fierce. Only the most skilled clinicians—those with self-awareness and knowledge—will succeed. This model has one fundamental intent: ideal results for both the clinician and the patient.

This *reference text* begins with chapters on the self and the team, then expands this knowledge to the patient-clinician relationship and creating positive outcomes. To this effect, general knowledge is expanded on, and insightful hints and recommendations allow you to optimize your knowledge and achieve the optimal, replicable results that will ensure your success. Each chapter has review questions and "Top Ten Tips to Take to the Clinic," which will help you well beyond your training and give you the knowledge that is helpful well beyond the classroom.

Good Luck!

About the Author

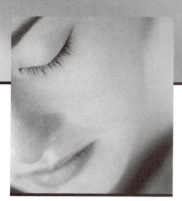

Pamela Hill, RN, CEO, received her diploma from Presbyterian/St. Luke's Hospital and Colorado Women's College. She followed through to practice as a registered nurse for more than 20 years with her initial emphasis in cardiac surgery and then in cosmetic surgery and medical skin care. In 1992, Ms. Hill founded Facial Aesthetics®, a network of medical skin care clinics in association with John A. Grossman, MD. Since then, Ms. Hill has been an industry pioneer in the growth and development of the medical spa industry. As the president and chief executive officer of Facial Aesthetics®, Ms. Hill has been a proactive member and pioneer in the evolution of the medical spa model and the integration and union of cosmeceuticals and nonsurgical skin care. In addition to her leadership in the medical spa industry, she has also been actively engaged in the research and development of the successful Pamela Hill Skin Care product line.

Ms. Hill has devoted her passion for nonmedical skin care to the instruction of a higher level of education and skill for those aspiring to be the aestheticians of tomorrow. To further this mission, Ms. Hill founded the Pamela Hill Institute® in 2004. The goal of the Pamela Hill Institute® is to develop a uniform and comprehensive curriculum, as well as provide resources for aesthetic education, the advancement of cutting-edge technologies, while placing an emphasis on client care and safety for patients, students, and product lines as well.

Reviewers

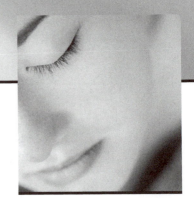

The author and publisher wish to thank the reviewers for their assistance and expertise in producing this text. We are indebted to them.

Darlene Battaiola,
Butte, Massachusetts

Alan Bunting,
Loxahatchee, Florida

Pat Cavenaugh,
Carolina Beach, North Carolina

Sallie Deitz,
Bellingham, Washington

Patricia Heitz,
Albany, New York

Ruth Ann Holloway,
Providence, Utah

Rose Policastro,
Little Ferry, New Jersey

Ellen Thorpe,
Mesa, Arizona

Karen Wackerman,
Phoenix, Arizona

Acknowledgments

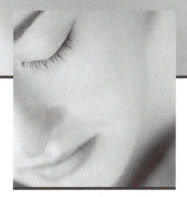

The Milady's Aesthetician Series is a group of books that will help clinicians grow to a new level. As the president and chief executive officer of a multilocation medical spa, I know how important this information is to our industry. I would like to acknowledge all of the aestheticians, nurses, and physicians assistants who strive each day to make a better place in our world.

I would also like to acknowledge the love of my life, my husband John. Always at my side, he has helped me to learn the skills of self-awareness, compassion, and what it means to provide superior patient care.

I would also like to acknowledge the staff at all of my clinics who supported me, taught me, and rallied me on to the goal line. However, there is one individual at my clinics that stands out, my regional manager, Pam Whatcott. She lessened my day-to-day worries about my clinics and took care of any and all problems, allowing me to focus on writing this book. Without her support and encouragement, this book would still be in the computer.

Additional thanks go to the people at Milady who believed in my message of advanced education and supported me through this process.

Milady and the author would like to thank the following for contributing to this series:

Larry Hamill Photography, Denver, CO

The owner, Edit Viski-Hanka, and her entire staff at Edit Euro Spa in Denver, CO, for allowing us to use their beautiful location for our photo shoot.

Aesthetic Technologies for graciously allowing the use of the Parisian Peel® Prestige™

Models who participated in the photo shoot:

Jessica Anderson Barbour	Julie O'Toole
Marnie Brooks	Jeffrey Robison
Tina Marie Castillo	Melissa Ryan
Beverley J. Grant	Kathryn Staples
Velma Guss	Christian M. Sterling
Alysa K. Hill	Kavina Trujillo
Patricia Iannacito	Lawrence P. Trujillo, Jr.
Rosalyn Kurpiers	Nina Tucciarelli
Sandra D. Martinez	Karyn Turner
Connee McAllister	Phyllis Walsh
Patricia J. McIntyre	Pamela Whatcott
Polly McKibben	Lisa Williams
Barbara J. Miller	Donna R. Wilson
Susan Nathan	Sandra Vinnik
Janene T. Newell	Edit Viski-Hanka

Social Perceptions

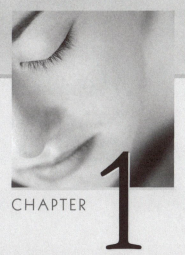

CHAPTER 1

KEY TERMS

adaptation	id	perception
character	individual	prejudice
ego	individual needs	psychology
fictional finalism	inferiority	social atomism
functional needs	integration	society
goal attainment	latencies	sociology
human condition	paradigm	superego

LEARNING OBJECTIVES

After completing this chapter you should be able to:

1. Discuss competing theories of individual and societal paradigms.
2. Identify the needs of the individual, as well as the needs of society.
3. Explain why tension exists between the individual and society.
4. Understand why these concepts are important for aesthetic practice.

INTRODUCTION

In most disciplines that use science as their basis, procedures and outcomes would ideally be straightforward. The patient is wounded, the wound gets treated, and the patient heals. In reality, however, things are never black and white (Figure 1–1).

Although we have made great strides in the diagnosis and treatment of many ailments, any physician or nurse would tell you that they treat people, not diseases. The major distinction, the gray area, is the considerations that intersect with the treatment. How a patient feels is inextricably linked to every step of the process, especially if the outcome has an effect on how the patient looks, feels, or is perceived by others. If the ultimate goal is an improvement in how the patient feels, positive outcomes cannot be achieved without knowing how, and fundamentally why, a patient feels throughout each step (Figure 1–1).

In the field of aesthetics, we straddle the fence between the social and the medical sciences. We use our knowledge of medicine to enhance the way people look, which has a notable effect on how people view themselves, as well as how other people view them. Therefore, when we consider the outcomes of these procedures, we, by necessity, must look at some of the social effects and consequences of the procedures we perform. Although this examination is certainly not the only consideration for achieving optimal outcomes, it is one with as much variability as significance. Furthermore, the psychosocial aspect is fairly fixed and one over which we have little leverage.

In the field of aesthetics, however, optimal outcomes will lay in your comprehension and compassion of patients' feelings rather than your ability to change them. Key to understanding why people feel one thing or another is thought to be the product of how individuals and the society in which they live interact with one another.

Understanding the **human condition** and how it interfaces with **society** is a complex study of social sciences. Some of the areas we will be discussing include concepts from **psychology** to **sociology** to communication; and although interesting, we will only be able to scan the surface of these subjects, preferring to use the concepts that apply to our

human condition
The situation of being human.

society
An organized group of persons: religious, scientific, political, or otherwise.

psychology
The science of the mind.

sociology
The study of human organizations.

Treatment Without Adequate Patient Consideration

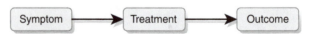

Figure 1–1   Treatment without consideration for the patient's psychologic and psychosocial priorities.

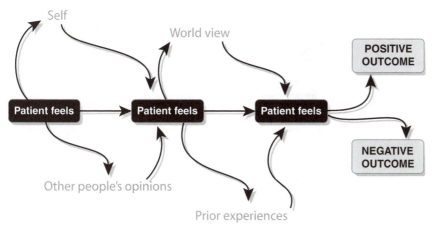

Figure 1–2   Treatment with consideration for the patient's psychologic and psychosocial priorities.

discussion of medical aesthetics rather than a thorough exploration of the subject matters.

▪ INDIVIDUAL

Several competing theories seek to explain the **individual** and that which motivates him or her. Although interesting, a complete discussion would certainly fill a text in its own right; but, a brief discussion is necessary because it is relevant to the practice of aesthetics. Two dominant theories in the social sciences are worth mentioning for our purposes.

The first theory was initially proposed by Sigmund Freud. According to him, the individual is guided mostly by unconscious forces. Freud used the interactions of the **id**, the **ego**, and the **superego** to explain the individual's motivations. The id represents primitive human desires to satisfy basic urges, such as those associated with hunger and sex. On the opposite end of the spectrum, the superego, is the moral and societal conscience as learned by the individual over time. Both the id and the superego represent the extreme positions, without a realistic assessment of time or place. This area is the buffer provided by the ego. The ego makes decisions by prioritizing urges and evaluating when and how best to act on them, given a particular situation.

For the aesthetician, this interaction might be evident as a patient or prospective patient weighs his or her personal desire to look better against preconceived notions of, for example, vanity or self-indulgence.

individual
A single human being.

id
The unconscious psyche; seeking pleasure.

ego
The "I" of someone.

superego
The conscience, formed early in life at the direction of parents and other behavioral role models.

inferiority
Less than.

fictional finalism
The perfect self as described by Adler.

paradigm
A model or pattern.

character
The features or traits of an individual.

perception
Cognitive awareness or recognition.
What the patient thinks of you.

"It has been said that man is a rational animal. All my life I have been searching for evidence that could support this."[2]
—*Bertrand Russell*

"What we *are* communicates far more eloquently than anything *we say or do*."[3]
—*S. R. Covey*

A second theory was first proposed by Alfred Adler, who split with the thinking of Freud because he believed the individual operated on a more deliberate and conscious level. He proposed that every person is striving to overcome **inferiority**. To this avail, each person has a general idea as to his or her perfect self, which Adler dubbed as ideal, "**fictional finalism**."[1] Furthermore, Adler theorized that our conscious and subconscious work in cohesion toward a realization of the fictional finalism. Complicating matters, individuals' nearly unattainable (and growing exponentially) fictional finalism qualities keep us always desiring to be better.

For the aesthetician, Adler's theories may be expressed in patients whose personal desires toward personal perfection have encompassed a need to look better and feel better. For most people, this expression is healthy; however, it may also be indicative of compulsive disorders that will require further investigation.

How the Individual Is Viewed by Society

As part of the human experience, we each have a unique set of experiences, circumstances, and beliefs that were shaped, in part, by upbringing, education, religious beliefs, and political beliefs. This unique perspective, or **paradigm**, defines our **character** and acts as a lens through which we view individuals and society. This paradigm sets the stage for our collective conflict: adapting the individual to be compatible with society, or vice versa, depending on the individual's scope. Either way, how we view and what we expect from one another is a key component to understanding the motivations of individual clients and the society at large.

Outward expressions of our characters create a **perception** of who we are to others and our place in the world. The ability to have *character greatness*[4] is the secret of give and take. The greatness is in the ability to give more than you receive and to make the giving come first. The concept seems simple, but in practice, it is not simple at all.

The lens through which we look also precipitates which groups with which we most identify, which groups we oppose, and which groups we belong or seek to belong. The opinions we have, or the indifference in some cases, are shaped by many factors, including many of the same ones that helped shape our character. For instance, someone whose character was greatly influenced by morality of the church would be likely to have close connections with religious institutions such as the church or church groups. These concepts, in fact, create our perceptions of the world; we see things objectively and as they are right *to us*. Based on our personal paradigm, we have opinions of certain groups of people, and these opinions can sometimes get in our way.

Prejudice is "an unfavorable opinion"[5] and can come in two types: love prejudice and hate prejudice. We are most familiar with hate prejudices. Prejudices are developed based on our "in-group-out-group" perceptions. Love prejudices come from believing the virtues of your in-group. Hate prejudices, on the other hand, come from identifying the "evil" of the out-group.[6] Prejudices and perceptions are powerful thinking and create paradigms that are unthinkable. Our perceptions—first impressions—are lasting impressions.

As we further investigate how we view the individual, we are not delving into each individual's personal beliefs or thought structures, but rather, the commonalities that may (or may not) influence how we collectively view the individual. This process is not as easy as it sounds. Let us refer to the authorities on the matter and go from there.

If a person were to ask Freud, he would say that the average individual is one half beast and one half civilized. As such, each of us is involved in a complex battle within ourselves. Our ego is constantly trying to integrate the primitive urges with the demanding mores imposed by a polite society. The stronger of the two forces (the id or the superego) deciphers the degree to which he or she will integrate into society.

Adler would emphasize the manner in which we approach the realization of our fictional finalism and overcoming inferiority. Adler believed that humans were one of four most common "types": the ruling types try to control others, the getting types are passive and go along with others, the avoiding types isolate themselves to avoid defeat, and the socially useful types embrace their individuality and do well for others as a means of improving society.

Regardless of the perspective with which you agree, if any at all, the important part to glean from this discussion is an understanding that, as individuals, we have certain needs that are expressed in a variety of ways. In general, each person has sought your services and counsel as a means to an end. Although you may agree or disagree with your patients' goals, knowing what has brought each client to see you will benefit you as an aesthetician.

Needs of the Individual

On the individual level, we act on our own behalves. Our decisions—and our actions—are usually motivated by a need to fulfill our own **individual needs**, wants, and goals. However, our goals may include acts of unselfishness, doing for others. Consider some of the volunteer activities that you may have done in the past or a random act of kindness

prejudice
An unfavorable opinion.

individual needs
Single human's necessities.

"A great many people think they are thinking when they are merely rearranging their prejudices."[7]
—*William James* (1842-1910)

Ensuring an optimal outcome is part education, part communication, and part execution.

you performed. Anyone who has done as much can identify with the feelings of gratification associated therein. On a bigger scale, the more people include the needs of others in their own set of needs, the greater the society will be on the whole. With this concept in mind, it would be safe to say that the needs of the individual are intertwined with the needs of society.

Abraham Maslow, an early twentieth century social scientist, devised a hierarchy of needs. He suggests the most basic needs are physiologic in nature. Above this basic level are the needs pertaining to safety, love, self-esteem, and self-actualization. The crux of his theory is that humans are motivated by unmet needs. The lower-level needs must be met before the higher needs can be met. Humans grow out of love. Maslow believed humans do not like violence, hate, or war. However, when the lower needs are not met, the human is usually destined to a life of violence, hate, or war. If humans do not feel safe, then war or violence become likely, despite the dislike of such. As human beings, we have an intrinsic need for purpose and a need to belong.

■ SOCIETY

Society is, in the most general of its purposes, the "body of institutions and relationships within which a relatively large group of people live."[8] In practice, society amounts to an organizational structure, in which "a plurality of individual actors interacting with each other in a situation which has at least a physical or environmental aspect, actors who are motivated in terms of a tendency to the 'optimization of gratification' and whose relation to their situations, including each other, is defined and mediated in terms of a system of culturally structured and shared symbols."[9] A debate exists in the social science circles over the significance of the notion of society. A noted sociologist, Emile Durkheim, took the position that society is the objective and that individuals are meant to do their part to contribute to societal perfection. Conversely, **social atomism** or methodologic individualism, first theorized by a Renaissance era philosopher named Thomas Hobbes, argued that society amounts to the sum of its many dynamic parts. Effectively, society as a dominant and determining body does not exist.

social atomism
Organizational elements.

How Society Is Viewed by the Individual

To sustain itself, society requires the active participation and benefits from those who meet their obligation. For the individual to be compelled to contribute on a grand scale, the rewards for successful contribution to the machine must be great enough to motivate or satisfy nearly all individual parts enough to perform day in and day out. As an example, a business will compensate persons under its employ with a significant contribution toward attaining their individual needs. This compensation may outwardly include salary and benefits but also reaches to areas such as shelter, safety, and other primitive needs of human beings. The same applies on the macroscopic level as well. In exchange for paying taxes—and maintaining the peace—society provides security, infrastructure, and institutions intended to ease the fulfillment of individuals' needs.

Just as the id and superego are juxtaposed, so are the individual and society. Each one is taking what they can, quid pro quo. In as much, a duality is inherent to this co-dependant relationship. Each one needs the other to perform a minimal set of obligations to sustain each other. Failure to deliver by either party would prove a catastrophic end for one or both.

In the aesthetic arena, society's influence is felt from two sides. The first side is more likely to be visible in the clinical setting. The influence is in the dynamic of an individual's need for societal approval, or the opposing expression, an individuals need to improve his or her self-image by outward progress. The appropriateness of either is not important in this context, however, it is worth mentioning again: determining a patient's suitability for treatment must be conducted on a singular basis. Second, and less of a presence, is the influence of how society at large views the aesthetics industry or the services they provide, or both. Although acceptance is nearly universal, certain sects dispel the benefits of, or even discourage acts of, beauty. With local exceptions, this group expresses a minority viewpoint with diminishing influence. Therefore the views of this group's members should have little bearing on society and the individuals involved.

Needs of Society

Social atomism involves an attractive sense of individualism toward which most self-determined people are drawn. However, one cannot ignore the organizational benefits society perpetuates. Imagine going door to door to take up a collection for street repairs. To accomplish this task, society has **functional needs**. These needs are **adaptation** (an economy to allocate resources), **goal attainment** (a political system to define societal objectives), **integration** (religion to symbolize moral unity and perpetuate solidarity among individuals), and **latencies** (primary and secondary associations to motivate individuals to perform their roles).[10]

> "Man is not made for society, but society is made for man. No institution can be good which does not tend to improve the individual."
> —*Margaret Fuller* (1810-1850)
> American social reformer

functional needs
The needs that cause a society to exist.

adaptation
An adjustment to cultural surroundings.

goal attainment
A term used to define objectives.

integration
The act of bringing together.

latencies
A stage of development, present but not visible.

You may wonder how does this discussion relate to you as the clinician. To be an effective clinician, and to ensure an optimal outcome for yourself and your patient, you will need to be adept at evaluating the functional needs on a case-by-case basis with each patient (adaptation), performing at your best (attainment), at times, counseling your patient as the progress (integration), all while satisfying your own goals and those of the clinic as well (latency).

Tensions Between the Individual and Society

When we speak of the needs of societies, the concepts of order and rules or laws apply. When we talk about the members of the society, the concepts of working interdependence and social responsibility resonate. However, individual personalities, beliefs, prejudices, and characters can sometimes be juxtaposed with the requirements of orderly society; hence tension can develop between the society and the individual.

Orderly societies can be identified throughout history. However, some of the most important qualities of the orderly society can be described only by the individuals who live within the society and their principles. Both society and the individual have unique and independent needs. This notion of need alone is not inherently bad, but because of the interdependent nature of this relationship, including "back-burner" or "what if" rationalizing (does an equal balance exist between resources expended and compensation received), it might seem as though both the individual and the society are hanging on but willing to jump ship for something better if and when it may arise.

■ PRACTICAL APPLICATION: CLINIC AND SPA AS A SOCIETAL MICROCOSM

All of this information is interesting, but how does it apply to the clinician? While describing the abstract concepts of the individual, we used the examples of individuals and their civic affiliations. However, a society can also include a much smaller entity, including your place of employment. Let us see how the place of employment being a medical aesthetic clinic (society) and the employee (individual) interact.

Clinician as the Individual

Earlier, we discussed two different theories that describe individuals and that which motivates them. Let us take this concept a step further and examine what motivates the clinician and how this may or may not contribute to an optimal outcome.

According to Freud, the clinician is guided by mostly unconscious forces. The id, which explains the more general or primitive motivations, may want to acquire money and benefits or to practice the skills that he or she has invested a great deal of time, effort, and sacrifice to attain. The superego will always be variant on the individual, given that these motivations have a moral basis. Some of these motivations might include a desire to help people or a need to be a valued team member. The ego, the conscious decision maker, enables the clinician to make moment decisions and practice his or her skills.

Conversely, if we looked at Adler's theory, the clinician is trying to overcome an inferiority. For instance, he or she had bad skin as an adolescent, or he or she wants to achieve greater financial stability than was the case before embarking on the training. The fictional finalism in these instances might be to either help make sure other adolescents have a better treatment option that will spare them ridicule or to have the financial security to travel or pay for a child's education, respectively.

Obviously, these examples are general in nature. As a student of aesthetics, you may want to evaluate your own motivations. Ask yourself, "Why do I want to be an aesthetician?" "What goals do I hope to achieve in doing so?" "How will I achieve said goals?"

Once you have answered these questions, you will have a better understanding of how you may view your clinic. The clinic (society) is your necessary means to meet your needs.

Clinic as a Society

As discussed, the perpetuation of the society depends on the willingness of the individual clinicians to work toward the collective goal of the organization. To reach this goal, the clinics offer their employees compensation. Compensation includes salaries, benefits, supplying necessary implements, and finding a location where the services can be performed. Similarly, the clinic has the ability to impose rules that dictate policy, behavior, and ethical standards to promote order and continuity. These steps are necessary to achieve the clinic's goal of financial solvency or public respect (Table 1–1).

Table 1–1   Functional Needs of the Clinic

Need	Definition	Example
Adaptation	An economy to allocate resources	Revenue
Goal attainment	Political system to define societal objectives	Hierarchy (e.g., managers, administrative staff, registered nurses, aestheticians)
Integration	Means of achieving moral unity and solidarity	Code of ethics, training procedures
Latencies	Secondary associations	Professional associations

Tensions Between the Clinic and the Clinician

As discussed, the clinic will offer the clinician compensation in exchange for adherence to company policy and a code of conduct. As is often the case, aspects that you find unpleasant about your place of employment may exist; for example, procedures, dress codes, or maybe another employee rubs you the wrong way.

You will be constantly evaluating whether these conflicts are so disruptive that they impede your ability to achieve your needs. The level of conflict will also vary from one individual to the next. However, nearly all persons would agree that their perception of the clinic (society) will be determined by the degree to which they enable your goals, above and beyond the distractions. Similarly, if the clinic itself perpetuates an environment with high turnover rates and frequent tensions, it is compromising its solvency.

Conclusion

The specific details of the dynamic between society and the individual have consequences and benefits in the aesthetics industry. The clinic, the patient, and the clinician are engaged in a delicate dance with one another. If one side of this dynamic fails to achieve its individual needs, the domino effect will be caustic for the other side. To achieve an optimal outcome, an awareness of all the needs, and how those needs relate to your own, is essential.

❱❱❱ TOP TEN TIPS TO TAKE TO THE CLINIC

1. Our life experiences mold our view of the world and ourselves.
2. What we say gives impressions of who we are and what we do.
3. Prejudices are unfair opinions that should be avoided at all costs.
4. Patients, similar to you, have their paradigm of the way they view the world.
5. Clinicians must be able to understand different paradigms and different opinions to be effective for and with patients.
6. Individuals are the "parts" of society and are dependent on society.
7. Maslow's principles still apply today and in our work.
8. Understand how you fit into the "clinical society."
9. There is a normal tension between a society and the individual.
10. Learn how to reassure patients in a positive and realistic manner.

CHAPTER REVIEW QUESTIONS

1. What is your individual paradigm of values and self?
2. Who constitutes the individual? Who comprises society?
3. What are the reasons that you believe that (a) societal betterment is the purpose of our individual pursuits or (b) society does not exist but rather is merely a collection of situational and ideologically similar individuals going about their affairs?
4. What tension exists in the dynamics between the individual and society?
5. What are prejudices? Do you have any prejudices that might influence your work? How would you define being empathic to the patient? Is empathy the same as compassion?
6. Why is Maslow's theory important to understand when you are working with patients?

BIBLIOGRAPHY

Covey, S. R. (1989). *The 7 habits of highly effective people.* New York: Simon and Schuster.

Lavington, C., & Losee, S. (2001). *You've only got three seconds.* New York: Broadway Books.

Merriam-Webster's Collegiate Dictionary. (1992). New York: Random House.

Moore, E. (Ed.). (1999). *Quotation finder*. Glasgow, Scotland: Harper Collins.

Parsons, T. (2005, May 24). *The social system*. [Online]. Available: http://www.mdx.ac.uk

Trinity University. (2005, January 29). *Social factors shaping perceptions and decision making*. [Online]. Available: http://www.trinity.edu

Williams, R. (1976). *Keywords: A vocabulary of culture and society*. New York: Fontana.

CHAPTER REFERENCES

1. Southern Methodist University. (2005, June 10). *Alfred Adler*. [Online]. Available: http://www.people.smu.edu

2. Moore, E. (Ed.). (1999). *Quotation finder*. Glasgow, Scotland: Harper Collins.

3. Covey, S. R. (1989). *The 7 habits of highly effective people*. New York: Simon and Schuster.

4. Covey, S. R. (1989). *The 7 habits of highly effective people*. New York: Simon and Schuster.

5. *Merriam-Webster's Collegiate Dictionary*. (1992). New York: Random House.

6. Trinity University. (2005, January 29). *Social factors shaping perceptions and decision making*. [Online]. Available: http://www.trinity.edu

7. Trinity University. (2005, January 29). *Social factors shaping perceptions and decision making*. [Online]. Available: http://www.trinity.edu

8. Williams, R. (1976). *Keywords. A vocabulary of culture and society*. New York: Fontana.

9. Parsons, T. (2005, May 24). *The social system*. [Online]. Available: http://www.mdx.ac.uk

10. Parsons, T. (2005, May 24). *The social system*. [Online]. Available: http://www.mdx.ac.uk

Strategies to Enhance Professional Relationships

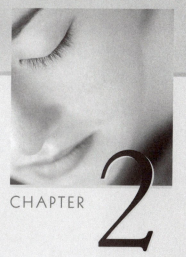

CHAPTER 2

LEARNING OBJECTIVES

After completing this chapter you should be able to:

1. Introduce the concepts of listening and active listening.
2. Explore different strategies for listening.
3. Discuss the different types of communication.
4. Learn the different components of communication.
5. Discuss how communication with co-workers and clients will help performance.

INTRODUCTION

From the moment we wake up to the moment we go to sleep, we exchange tens of thousands of words with people. Without the ability to do so, living in a social and orderly manner would be quite difficult. We need to communicate with one another for many reasons, of varying importance. Every part of our bodies, our senses, our voices, and our gestures are engaged in a perpetual transmission of verbal and nonverbal codes from which we send and receive information, assign value levels, and retain (or discard) information. In similar situations, different people will assign different levels of importance to the same piece of information. Pointing, for example, is a common form of communication in our culture; in other cultures, it is considered offensive.

In aesthetics, the degree to which we can or cannot communicate can have far-reaching implications. These implications extend to the client's well being, your livelihood (not to mention the livelihood of your co-workers), and the overall success of the business. Failing to read signals, hear important details, and act in accordance will certainly have a bearing on the outcome of any procedure.

Furthermore, in the field of aesthetics, a triangular relationship exists among the patient, yourself, and the clinic. Your role will be paramount in this relationship because you will often be the go-between for the clinic and the patient. You will need to act as an advocate and a representative when interacting on the other one's behalf. As such, exploring the different avenues of communication will make you better prepared for clinical practice, as well as most other life situations.

■ TYPES OF COMMUNICATION

communication
The transmission of information by use of symbols.

Communication is the use of symbols to relay information. Some of these symbols involve words, some involve expression, some use gesturing, and some involve a combination of all forms. Contrary to what some people may believe, communication does not necessarily involve receiving. If you ask for directions from a person on the road, you have communicated with that person. Now, suppose you are in another country, and you do not speak the same language as the other person on the road. Did you not communicate your need for directions, even though he or she did not understand? Consider advertising. If a commercial comes on the radio, you either listen or tune it out. The advertiser has still communicated its product or event. The mere act of sending the information is communicating. Receiving information is a different matter, discussed later. First, let us examine how information is sent.

Animal Communication

Humans are not the only beings who communicate. Nearly all animals use sounds to communicate with one another. Although much less understood, animals also use nonverbal communication cues as well. Cross-species communication is rare but not uncommon. For example, humans and their pets are capable of communicating basic needs and emotions. Similarly, animals will rely on other animals to garner information. An example of this type of communication would be land-dwelling animals reacting to the behavior of birds in the sky or the movement of leaves on a tree to indicate the presence of a predator or natural disaster.

Telecommunication

We tend to think of technology or machinery when we think of telecommunications. Rather, telecommunications is the sending of information over large areas of space, as is the case with mass media (such as television, radio, and film) or even smoke signals. Any form of communication that is sent to a multiplicity of persons who are separated by a distance that would make ordinary interpersonal communication ineffective is considered telecommunication.

Interpersonal Communication

Interpersonal communication, also called dyadic communication, involves communication between one person to another. This type of communication usually involves listening, dialog exchange, summarizing, paraphrasing, and gesturing. A greater instance of reception exists in this form of communication compared with other types. However, the substance of the communication may not be the information the sender intended. Interpersonal communication uses both verbal and nonverbal methods.

Verbal Communication

Most often, we use words and language to send information. When a potential sender has a thought or an **idea**, the **verbal communication** has its berth. For the receiver to understand the message, the information needs to be encoded. **Encoding** is a cognitive process by which the sender organizes ideas into symbols. People who are adept at verbal communication will take steps to ensure that the intended recipient

interpersonal communication
Also called dyadic communication, involves communication between one person to another.

idea
The beginning step of communication. Concepts and thoughts are translated into symbols and sent to the intended receiver.

verbal communication
Type of interpersonal communication that involves the use of symbols, particularly words and other sounds, to send information to a recipient.

encoding
Part of communication that deals with translating ideas into symbols, such as words or letters, to best enable the receiver's understanding.

internal noises

Any distractions from within, such as
wondering or closed mind, that inhibit
the understanding of a sent message.

external noises

Any outside distractions that interfere
with the comprehension of a sender's
message.

**nonverbal
communication**

A type of interpersonal communication
whereby the sending of a message is
accomplished without a verbal cue. This
task is usually accomplished with hand
signals, gesturing, posturing, and eye
movements.

understands the message. To accomplish this task, words, actions, and
tone are considered and chosen with the recipient in mind. The message
is decoded and received.

Verbal communication also involves the use of inflection and
volume to send a message. If a person is talking in loud tones, it conveys
a different meaning than if the message is said in a low, monotone
fashion.

No matter how well or accurately a message is encoded, **internal
noises** and **external noises** complicate matters. Senders and receivers
experience internal noise. How they perceive the topic will affect how
the sender packages the message and how the receiver interprets it.
External noise, the environmental factors of traffic, competing conversation, or even hearing loss, can also interfere.

Nonverbal Communication

Nonverbal communication is the process of sending a message without a verbal cue. Although nonverbal communication is usually perceived as "no," it can sometimes mean "yes." The most common
nonverbal communication involves the use of facial expressions. Try to
remember that old expression, "the eyes are the window to the soul."
Your eyes are the most powerful nonverbal communicator. Your eyes
can tell others what you are thinking: if you believe in yourself, or if you
believe the product you recommend has value. Hand gestures, body
movements, touch, and personal space also play a role in nonverbal
communication. Silence itself can sometimes convey information. If you
are talking during a class and your instructor stops talking and stares at
you, you would easily ascertain the need for you to pay attention.

Hand gestures are an important nonverbal communication tool. If
you are not accepting or open to ideas, you may be bored, thus folding
your arms in front of you. Additionally, folded arms, theoretically, also
reflect a closed mind. Tapping fingers and fidgeting with your finger-
nails are negative nonverbal communication cues. Furthermore, touching others is a nonverbal cue. A common touching technique is the
squeeze of a hand or arm to offer reassurance. Similarly, using hand gestures can be used to emphasize or expand on verbal communication.
Someone saying something while pounding his or her fist is meant to
emphasize the words or the emotion of the speaker. If someone is talking
about the shape of a circle, drawing one in the air would be more helpful
than explaining that it is a "closed plane curve everywhere equidistant
from a given, fixed center."[1]

Body movements can also convey a meaning, whether implied or
not, whether intentional or not. If someone is sitting slouched, with his

or her head rested, you might assume that the person is tired; or if you wanted to demonstrate respect, you may stand up when someone enters a room. Even the way you posture yourself while walking, sitting, or speaking says something in accordance with, or in opposition to, the words you use. Some people use these nonverbal cues more than using the words themselves. How you posture yourself can tell someone how much you believe what you are saying, if you are lying, or if you know the subject you are discussing. Self-image also plays a part in nonverbal communication. How you feel about yourself and your message will be reflected in your nonverbal cues.

Touch and personal space are important. Everyone has had the experience of being in an elevator when it is packed with people. Being that close to people whom you do not know can be an uncomfortable experience. Have you ever been talking to someone, and they move closer to you than is comfortable? Give people their space, and respect their need to have distance from you when you talk. Someone who is right in your face while they are talking can have a specific meaning. In our culture, this gesture expresses anger, or it is an intimidation mechanism. In other cultures, standing close to the person to whom you are talking is considered friendly or respectful. Similarly, touch can imply affection or aggression, depending on the degree on pressure applied.

■ LISTENING

Do you know what it means to really listen? **Listening** is not just hearing what another person says; it is an active process of understanding what the other person is saying, even if the person does not verbally say so. Listening involves the translation of verbal and nonverbal cues to extrapolate a meaning that the speaker wants to convey. Although some people are direct in what they mean or how they feel, others have difficulty in expressing themselves. Further complicating matters, in different situations, the degree to which we listen varies. Suppose you are on a date with someone to whom you are attracted. You might be hanging on to every word and attempting to gauge compatibility. Chances are that you would be able to remember the smallest detail much later. Now suppose you were on a blind date with someone with whom the attraction was minimal. You might be wondering if you will be home in time to watch the evening news. Our degree of **active listening** varies greatly with the importance of the information being offered. When the information has greater personal meaning, we will be engaged in more active listening.

In the clinical setting, the information being offered is of great importance to you and to the patient who gives the information. As mentioned, listening and hearing what the other person is saying are not one in the

listening
An active process of understanding what a sender is meaning, even if the person does not verbally say so. Listening involves the translation of verbal and nonverbal cues to extrapolate a meaning.

active listening
The process by which the receiver of information is paying attention to verbal and nonverbal cues as a means to understand fully the message the sender intends.

listening strategies
The use of different types of listening to keep your focus while extracting the information you are intended to garner.

top-down listening strategy
The listener uses background knowledge on the subject or the person for the purpose of listening for main ideas, predicting, drawing conclusions, and summarizing.

bottom-up listening strategy
A listening strategy during which the receiver uses grammar and word choice to understand the intended message of the sender.

same. Good listening skills are learned and represent more than the process of just hearing words. Learning to be a good listener requires that you understand the concepts of active listening. People who are active listeners use what are called **listening strategies** to accomplish understanding. Employing these strategies will help you keep your focus while extracting the information you will need to ensure an optimal outcome.

Listening Strategies

Listening strategies can be divided into three types. In the first type, the **top-down listening strategy**, the listener uses background knowledge on the subject or the person for the purpose of listening for main ideas, predicting, drawing conclusions, and summarizing. This strategy is a valuable tool that many professionals use. However, it is not the best strategy to use, given the high probability for misinterpretation. When you scan the information that is being provided to you for points relative to your range of knowledge, you may be minimizing the other person's information as it relates to them.

Next is the **bottom-up listening strategy**. In this strategy, the listener uses the language and grammar to understand meaning. This method includes listening for specific details, recognizing cognates, and

Listening Strategy Techniques

To practice listening strategies, both in the clinical setting and beyond, things to do would include:

- Focus on the person who is talking. Look at him or her in the eye, and watch for gestures.
- Avoid distractions. Close the door and preserve silence.
- Be aware of your nonverbal communication and how it will affect the client.
- Be involved without taking over.
- Let the client finish what he or she is saying; do not interrupt.
- Ask questions that do not require yes or no answers; one-word answers will not allow the client to explore his or her concerns.
- Summarize the patient's feelings to be sure you have the whole picture.
- Do not assume.
- Do not give meaningless reassurances (e.g., "Oh, don't worry about it.")
- Reacting is acceptable as long as the reaction is appropriate and from a neutral paradigm.
- Remember, using the word "I" too much in speaking does not indicate good listening. If I do all of the talking, then how can I listen?

identifying specific word order patterns. This strategy would be ideal if everyone used language the same way with the same degree of mastery, which, unfortunately, is not always the case. A good example of this strategy is the use of the word *bad* in the affirmative.

The final strategy is called the **metacognitive listening strategy**. Metacognitive listeners are accomplished at using both bottom-up and top-down strategies. They can use both simultaneously and switch between both to garner the messages most effectively. They can plan on using the strategy that will be best served in a particular situation, monitoring their comprehension, and switching to another strategy if they believe their comprehension goals are not being met. For you, a future clinician, you will obviously be best served with the metacognitive strategy. However, you will need to practice top-down and bottom-up strategies first.

Listening and Empathy

Once you have become adept at the different types of listening strategies, you can start using some communication cues that will impart a sense of understanding to the person with whom you are communicating, primarily, **empathy**. Empathy is letting the talker know that his or her feelings and intentions are understood but not judged. As clinicians, we must be able to use skills that involve empathy, communicating to our patients that we understand and appreciate what they are saying and feeling. Being empathetic often communicates that the clinician *respects* the patient's views and feelings. The ability to be empathetic and respect the patient's views is a step in the process of problem solving. When the concepts of empathy and listening are wielded together, the clinician can help the patient by being a problem solver. Listening is a difficult skill to master. Being quiet and waiting for your turn to talk is difficult, especially if you like to talk. However, allowing the patient to speak and not be uninterrupted is a key to hearing his or her problems. The more you understand your patient's problems, and the effects that they have for the patient, the more likely you are to develop a trusting and lasting professional relationship (Table 2–1).

■ EFFECTIVE COMMUNICATION FOR THE AESTHETICIAN

As we have discussed, communicating and listening are active processes that will require the sender and the receiver to keep on their toes. Your success as a clinician will depend greatly on your ability to do so effectively. The treatment plans that you recommend for your clients

metacognitive listening strategy
Using of both top-down and bottom-up strategies simultaneously to garner the messages most effectively. Persons who use this strategy will be best served in a particular situation: they monitor their comprehension and switch to another strategy if they believe their comprehension goals are not being met.

empathy
Using thoughts, words, and actions as a means of conveying a deep level of understanding.

Webster's dictionary defines empathy as "the action of understanding, being aware of, being sensitive to, and vicariously experiencing the feelings, thoughts, and experience of another."[2]

Table 2–1   Characteristics of Empathy and Listening

Characteristics of Empathy	Characteristics of Good Listening
Put yourself in the speakers "shoes."	Focus on the speaker, not on yourself.
Respect the speaker.	Allow the speaker to complete his or her thoughts without interruption.
Be nonjudgmental.	Wait your turn.

will be successful only if you have fully comprehended what the patient's desired results are for treatment, as well as gauged the expectations for feasibility. However, the clear lines of communication should not be limited to those between clinician and client. Open and accurate channels of communication between the clinician and fellow team members within the clinic are also vital. This group includes other aestheticians, nurses, physicians, and ancillary staff.

Communication and Team Membership

Teams are strange beasts. They develop personalities and the ability to accomplish lofty goals when they are focused and *on target*. However, when teams are dysfunctional, nothing can be worse. The best teams are those that hold the same objectives and foster trust and safety, creating an environment to give opinions and participate freely. Team members must feel passionate about their work and the goals they hope to achieve. When team members share a common passion, meeting the objectives will come much easier. Anyone who works well with another should hold similar values with that person. The team anatomy should include not only the members, but also team leaders or management. This leader should be a respected member of the team who participates in a meaningful way to achieving a goal. Similarly, the team leader should be equally adept at relating to fellow teammates while being able to delegate properly to those most likely to produce the best outcome.

No doubt, many clinicians have experience in communicating with patients. In fact, some clinicians are good at it. However, communicating with physicians, nurses, and other professionals may be new to you and may pose additional challenges. Professional communication can carry physiologic baggage, such as a fear of authority figures, disrespect for *the establishment,* or simply being intimidated by the situation. To overcome some of these feelings, the clinician can take several steps. Listening is an important beginning! For the clinician to respond properly, he or she must understand what is being said. If you are new to the field, you might consider taking a notebook along when speaking with the physician or nurse. This approach will eliminate the panic of having forgotten the essence of the information when you return to your treatment room. When information is forgotten (and it can happen in the walk back to the treatment room), you will need to ask the questions again. This unfortunate incident will reflect poorly on you, making you appear unprepared or unprofessional. Additionally, having to ask the same questions again is a waste of time for everyone, the clinician included. Notes can also come in handy later when similar situations arise.

Step two is the process of restating. This process may seem silly and embarrassing, but it is the best way to ensure you have understood the information. Again, write down the information. Be attentive when your colleagues are speaking to you. Avoid sending negative body language or nonverbal communication that is unintended. In fact, this area is one that the medical spa clinician must fully understand. Negative body language and unintended nonverbal communication can be misinterpreted and reflect poorly on you. Finally, your turn comes to speak or respond. How something is said can be more important than what is said. Be sure that you are aware of the tone of your voice and your attitude. You want both to reflect positives!

If you are initiating a conversation with the physician about a patient, of critical importance is having your facts straight, which means that you can give the patient history, for example, with succinct

> For the clinician to respond properly, he or she must understand what is being said. Honing listening skills is the first step.

Poor Communication

Poor communication is the primary reason that health care often reaches an impasse. The inability to communicate clearly can often be blamed for the inability to provide the best health care. In the medical spa world, communication and coordination of the treatment plans are essential for a positive patient outcome. Some of the breakdown can come when multiple clinicians are taking care of the patient. Given that clinicians are really an extension and reflection of the physician, communication between the patient and the clinician and between the clinician and the rest of the staff must be clear and well documented.

accuracy. Nothing is more frustrating for a physician than a clinician who does not understand or know the patient history and cannot give a good understanding of the situation. If your purpose in speaking with the physician is, presumably, to ask his or her opinion or direction, be sure you have all the facts. Otherwise, you will look foolish, and you will be wasting the physician's time. These types of situations will make the physician or nurse lose confidence in you and your skills, ultimately affecting your ability to be successful in a medical environment. It may sound snobbish, but physicians like smart people. Remember, physicians have spent years in school and have been exposed to scholars and worldwide experts; their expectation is that you are also an expert in your field, which means you must also behave as a professional. Your standards must reflect that of the physician for whom you work and the field you have chosen.

Obstacles to Effective Communication

Obviously, effective communication has many components and requires an equaled effort by each involved party. This circumstance leaves a great deal of room for error, thus compromising the flow of information; it also leaves the patient, the clinicians, and the clinic as a whole susceptible to less-than-desirable consequences (Table 2–2). Although many obstacles can hinder communication, our emphasis will focus exclusively on the one that will have the greatest impact on clinical results: conflict.

Interrupting is a terrible habit; it is unprofessional and disrespectful. Think about it. Do you like to be interrupted? Does it cause you to lose your train of thought? Does it frustrate you? This habit falls squarely into the category of the "Golden Rule."

Table 2–2   Unintentional Nonverbal Communication

Negative Nonverbal Communication	Change to Make
Avoiding eye contact	Look directly at the person who is speaking.
Folding the arms across the chest	Clasp the hands in front or carry a notebook.
Tapping feet, pencil, or fingers	Be aware of and avoid doing this.
Closeness of personal space	Respect personal space.

If you are an interrupter, stop it. You must let the speaker finish! Interrupting can be incredibly frustrating for the speaker and creates an inconsistency in the flow of the conversation and the information being transmitted. If the compromised flow of conversation does not result in miscommunication, then the irritation it causes will. Repeated encounters with someone who interrupts will cause someone to either refuse to communicate or modify their means of communicating with the interrupter. Both of these mechanisms can impede the transmission of

Simple Ways to Avoid Malpractice

Our society holds physicians in high esteem. More is expected from physicians than from any other professional group. Our expectation is that they know *everything*, should be able to make *anything* better, and that they are *infallible*, meaning that they will cure us or save our loved one from pain and suffering.

As the number of malpractice cases rises, tort reform is a governmental priority. However, the physician is not perfect, and tort reform is slow in being perfected. Why then do we have this schism of reality as it relates to physicians? Do we really *expect* our physicians to know everything? Probably not. Important causes can be cited for the increase in malpractice claims. Aside from the patient-physician relationship, we should also consider increasing specialization, procedures offered, procedures performed by technicians (versus physicians), patient expectations that have been influenced by the media, an increase awareness of patient rights, the decline of physicians' public image, the government's involvement in medicine, and, finally, the increasing cost of medical care.[3] What patients *really* seem to want is a dose of compassion and elixir of time. The *Journal of the American Medical Association* recently published a study by the Agency for Health Care Policy regarding the patient-physician communication and malpractice suits. The study was randomized and controlled and found that when physicians talked to patients more—told patients what they were going to do, spent time with patients, elicited opinions and questions from patients, used appropriate humor, and laughed more—they were less likely (if at all) to have malpractice claims. Therefore should we just want our physicians to be people too? Well, yes and no. Being treated by a physician who is a poor practitioner but a great communicator would not be good enough. This circumstance certainly happens, but in the best cases, we want knowledgeable physicians who are just people too.

information. If you have a need to interrupt, write your thoughts down. However, if you usually let the speaker finish, your comments may become unimportant, or your question will be answered. In many cases, when someone is interrupted, his or her attention will be on the interruption rather than the words. When your message is valid, you need not talk over others or raise your voice.

When you are the speaker, do not talk too loudly. Speaking in a loud voice can be distracting to your message. The listener can be intimated by the volume of your voice, and the meaning of the message can change. Have you ever been yelled at when the message was not a *yelling* message?

Additionally, another situation that impedes communication and can cause conflict is not speaking to your audience. The best example of this situation is with teachers of young children. Given that teachers modify their inflections and word choices so often for their students, teachers will often do the same thing at inappropriate times, such as when they are talking with their peers or spouse. As an aesthetician, you will need to make sure that you do not "dumb down" your conversations with patients or with staff members. No one likes to feel as though they are intellectually inferior.

Conflict

Conflict presents a difficult situation for many people and exhibits behaviors that one would not normally expect from that particular individual. Some people protect themselves from conflict by yelling, and others choose not to participate. If you can, step away from the problem (do not run away), and try to evaluate the situation intellectually, not emotionally. People who approach conflict emotionally always lose something valuable, either their dignity or something economic. For example, when a new practice administrator comes into the facility, the rules can change. This change is sometimes met with conflict by staff members, and at other times, it is met as opportunity. Ineffective communication can be suspected when conflict arises.

Conflict will most often occur as a result of perceived opposing ideas. This situation can evolve a team to the next level, or it can tear the team apart. If ideas can be discussed, and if the best parts of all of the concepts can be used, the team will propel to the next level. If, on the other hand, you are married to your ideas and cannot discuss them without conflict, communication will usually fail. Ideas can be personal, and a perceived attack can create conflict of a personal nature. Clearly state your position and avoid an emotional response while actively listening to opposing ideas is the answer. This approach can usually lead the team to the right decision. Opposition is a fundamental component to collaboration when it is done constructively. If constructive criticism leads to conflict, then ineffective communication is almost certainly the cause.

Conflict Resolution

Conflict resolution is a science in and of itself. Depending on the conflict and the parties involved, conflict resolution can be accomplished easily between the persons involved, on one end of the spectrum, or it can lead to mediation or litigation on the opposite extreme. Most conflicts can be resolved quickly and effectively when the right communication skills are employed.

Resolving conflict is important for a team. Highly functioning teams are able to identify problems and work through them for the greater good of the team and its goals. In fact, some teams have such cohesion that they can accomplish conflict without even realizing that they are doing so. Resolution requires that all parties make an effort to talk through and improve the situation.

conflict resolution
The act of creating solutions to problems.

Conclusion

How do you put all of this information together and positively affect your position on the medical spa team? As a medical aesthetician, you are a member of a team that cares for patients. Your input is important to the overall care of the patient, and your opinions are valuable. Your ability to be a highly functioning member of the team ensures that your opinions and ideas will be heard. We have mentioned that you will be an agent of your patient's needs and your clinic. Being well adept at communicating with your patients, knowing when and how to seek advice or opinions, relaying that information to the appropriate staff members and the patient alike will depend on your ability to sort through a host of spoken words and unspoken rules. Taking the time to understand the fundamentals of communication will better prepare you for the delicate dance you will be doing as a medical aesthetician.

▶ ▷ ▷ TOP TEN TIPS TO TAKE TO THE CLINIC

1. Practice good listening skills.
2. Part of the physician's communication style is influenced by his or her individual histories, as well as their education.
3. Success in your career, especially in the medical spa, depends on your communication skills.
4. Nonverbal communication cues can be disruptive to your message.
5. Take notes when speaking to a physician or other staff members so you do not forget what was said.

6. Learn how to be a highly functioning member of the health care team.

7. Avoid interrupting, speaking out of turn, or speaking above the listener's knowledge of the subject.

8. Learn to manage your feelings so you can avoid communication conflict.

9. Conflict is part of the resolution process. Try to work through situations as they arise.

10. Make sure your ideas are heard. You are important.

CHAPTER REVIEW QUESTIONS

1. What is communication?
2. What are the types of communication?
3. What are the different components to interpersonal communication?
4. In what ways can communication be compromised?
5. What are the different communication styles that might make your patient care easier or harder?
6. Why are nonverbal communication cues important?
7. Why are your ideas important to the team?
8. What is listening? What are the differences between listening and active listening?
9. What are the three types of listening strategies? Why is one strategy better for aestheticians?

BIBLIOGRAPHY

Fox, Y. M. (1995). *The American Academy of Orthopaedic Surgeons bulletin* [Online]. Available: www.aaos.org

Merriam-Webster's Collegiate Dictionary. (1992). New York: Random House.

CHAPTER REFERENCES

1. *Merriam-Webster's Collegiate Dictionary.* (1992). New York: Random House.
2. *Merriam-Webster's Collegiate Dictionary.* (1992). New York: Random House.
3. Fox, Y. M. (1995). *The American Academy of Orthopaedic Surgeons bulletin* [Online]. Available: www.aaos.org

Ethics and Patient Rights

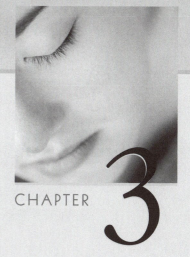

CHAPTER 3

KEY TERMS

consequentialist ethics
ethics
personal ethics

principled ethics
professional code of
  ethics

professional ethics
regulations
virtue ethics

LEARNING OBJECTIVES

After completing this chapter you should be able to:

1. Discuss and define ethics.
2. Understand your ethical role in the clinic.
3. Discuss the different types of ethics.
4. Explain the difference between personal and professional ethics.
5. Understand the importance of a professional code of ethics.

INTRODUCTION

We have discussed how communication and psychology play a role in developing and maintaining a relationship with your patients. We have defined some different theories therein, which will help you relate to and communicate with your patients. However, one more piece is needed to complete the core platform that will, ultimately and ideally, contribute to your professional success. Not only will you need to read, interpret, and communicate with your patients, but you will also need to employ the basic principles of **ethics** to achieve optimal outcomes for your patient and for yourself.

Acting in an ethical manner is a matter of importance for persons in the allied medical fields. The results of doing otherwise will affect your ability to create lasting relationships, ultimately jeopardizing your career. With so much riding on the subject, paying strict attention to the guidelines put forth by the industry itself, professional organizations, and your employer is to your advantage. You may also want to consider your own **personal ethics** to avoid conflicts between belief and practice. We will go deeper into this subject later in the chapter. However, first, let us start from the beginning. What are ethics?

ethics
Moral values or principles.

personal ethics
Personal values.

DEFINING ETHICS

Are ethics and success mutually exclusive? Do you need to be unethical to be successful, or the more ethical you are, the more successful you will be? Today, business schools are loaded with courses on the ethical behavior in the business world. One need to look only as far as companies such as Enron to seed the fertile ground for discussion. These examples demonstrate the darker side of unethical behavior. The behavior of a few people resulted in the loss of billions of dollars and thousands of jobs, destroying hundreds of lives. However, no one would have tried to pursue such acts if many more had not gotten away with it beforehand.

Unfortunately, the answer to these questions is rarely straightforward. In their most basic forms, ethical principles have their foundations in religion. Concepts found in the "Golden Rule," or the Ten Commandments for that matter, have been commonly used to create ethical statements. In fact, many of the ethics we use in business today find history in the tenets of organized religion.[1] However, in reality, ethics lie between law and punishment on one hand and religion or virtue and sin on the other.[2]

The dictionary tells us that ethics are "the body of moral principles or values held by or governing a culture, group or individual."[3] Until recently, our world rarely emphasized business ethics. The meaning of living an ethical life or working in an ethical environment was left to the individual, with boundaries set by the society. However, one cannot deny that corrupt management and the disparity in salaries between company employees and corporate executives of that same company begs us to look at ethics in the workplace.

If asked, each of you has a base of principles or ethics by which you live each day. You know the right thing to do, and when you consider the *wrong thing,* it ties your stomach in knots. However, these problems are seemingly easy to solve. What about the grayer issues that go on in the typical salon, day spa, or medical spa? Consider the following example. A client comes in on Wednesday for an eyebrow wax. You have never met her before. In the interview, she says she uses Retin A® regularly but over the last week has discontinued the product. She is getting married on Saturday and would like you to wax and shape her eyebrows. You agree to do so. During the procedure, you lift skin from both eyebrow areas. What seemed so simple is now complex. Did she really stop using her Retin A®? Does she use other products that might cause a problem? Did she offer any examples of previous experiences with waxing? Did you ask about previous experiences? Did you provide the procedure with the correct techniques? What do you do now? Do you refund her money? Give her a gift certificate? Did she accept part of the risk? She trusted that you would take good care of her, knowing she had a special event. Does this situation present an ethical dilemma? What is the right thing to do? Although we can wish for simple answers, none can be found, even in the most apparently easy situations.

To further distill the ideas of ethics and right versus wrong, we will employ three types of ethical theories: **virtue ethics, consequentialist ethics,** and **principled ethics**[4] (Table 3–1). Other variations of these formulas can be found, but for our purposes, we will simplify our discussion to these three. Each theory is limited by the definitions of the specific ethical concept. In other words, the definitions are narrow and may require overlap as you begin to use and understand the application. Additionally, understanding that ethics has different approaches and is not as simple as right versus wrong may help. Furthermore, these ethical strategies can be used for both personal ethics and **professional ethics**.

■ IMPORTANCE OF ETHICS

As far back as the time of Moses and the Ten Commandments, a guide has existed for right versus wrong. Nonetheless, even the Ten

virtue ethics
The principles of character.

consequentialist ethics
Psychologic traits; the outcome of the situation is most important.

principled ethics
Morals or principles that everyone should know and understand.

professional ethics
Guidelines of behavior for the professional.

Table 3–1   Three Ethical Theories

Ethical Theory	Ethical Definition
Virtue ethics	Focuses on character
Consequential ethics	Focuses on personality traits
Principled ethics	Focuses on right and wrong

Commandments require interpretation.[5] However, life was easier then. Less interpretation was necessary. The large cities of our world often put us in conflict with our ethics and values. In cities, we are exposed to more: more situations, more people, and more opportunities. Each new situation may force us to evaluate our ethics and personal values. These situations require reflection and evaluation, recognizing that "there is more than one way to skin a cat," as the old saying goes; and sometimes, more than one right and ethical answer exists. That said, not every situation is an ethical discussion, and knowing the difference is important.

Those of us who enter into a career of caring—a job that involves the lives of our patients each day—may face difficult situations from time to time. A patient will sometimes share information with us that forces us into uncomfortable circumstances that require evaluation of your ethics and perhaps a rethinking of our opinion based on a broad interpretation of the ethical theory. If the situation causes a knot in your stomach, you need to understand why, beyond "it just does not feel right." Just because the situation does not feel right does not mean that you have fairly analyzed the situation or, for that matter, that you are fairly applying the multiple theories of ethical interpretation. Furthermore, unknown prejudices can complicate the situation. Understanding feelings (ethics and ethical theory) and recognizing prejudices help make a balanced and fair decision. Let us look at a few examples.

Your patient is in the clinic for a treatment today and is in need of a cleanser. She has used a particular cleanser for quite some time, but you are out of that cleanser today. You have several other cleansers, one that is similar and one that is quite different. What is the right answer? Is this an ethical question or a simple business dilemma? Do you try to recommend a different cleanser, even though she is attached to the back-ordered brand? Do you simply give the facts and let the patient decide? What if she takes the recommended cleanser but then wants to return it in a week? What is right? What is wrong?

Consider this more difficult situation. Your patient is in the clinic from out of town. After her facial, she would like to have Botox®, but she is not on the schedule for Botox®. Your clinic usually buys only enough Botox® for the day. Apparently, a small amount will be available at the end of the day. What do you do? Do you tell the patient that the Botox® supply for her treatment is limited, and because she was not on the schedule, she will need to reschedule when she returns? Should you suggest that the nurse do a mild treatment because you are running low on the product? Should you say nothing at all? Given that she is leaving town first thing in the morning, you will miss the revenue if you do not do something. What is the right answer?

■ PERSONAL ETHICS

The foundation of personal ethics is usually tied to, or modified from, those of religious, traditional, and political beliefs. Some of our personal ethics are well known to us, whereas others are less known. Our ethics help us interpret which behaviors (for ourselves and others) are acceptable and which are not. Three types of ethical principles have been developed that we will discuss to assist us in categorizing the information we receive: virtue ethics, consequentialist ethics, and principled ethics. Virtue ethics is that of character. Are we *good people*, whatever that may mean? Those of us in caring careers usually have strong virtue ethics because relationships are important to us. Consequentialist ethics are those that derive a consequence, in other words, the ethical behavior or expected ethical behavior of a person in society and how the behavior of each person affects the society at large. Lastly, we will be talking about principled ethics. This type of ethics is an accepted school of thought about the situation. In other words, principled ethics are what the majority believes, and, as we know, this will change between groups and, on a larger scale, between cultures. Each theory has positive and negative components to its use. Moreover, all three concepts are usually a part of each person's personal ethical principles.

Virtue Ethics

Virtue ethics focuses on character,[6] the element of ethical questioning that looks at "what kind of person should I be?" These ethical principles are the ones that define our character as we see ourselves. They are rooted in our personal happiness and our personal definitions of success. Virtue ethics focuses on our goodness and ability to fulfill what it means to be a good person. This definition or model of ethics has a powerful place for those of us who entered our careers to *help people* or *make a difference for people*; it is the primary ethic instilled as a child. Parents will tell children "be nice to your friends, or they won't come back to play" or "it is a greater gift to give than to receive." Virtue ethics is a commonly discussed theory and one that we expect everyone should have in his or her inherit behaviors. Virtue ethics is also, in part, responsible for a smooth running society: volunteer work or *random acts of kindness*. These behaviors we consider *virtuous* are responsible, in part, for a smoothly functioning society.

Consequential Ethics

The second theory is called consequential ethics. This theory focuses on psychologic traits versus the personality traits of virtue ethics. In this ethical model, the outcome of the situation is more important than the person. In other words, the result is the indicator of ethics. Consequential ethics dictates which behavior will provide the greatest good for all involved. For example, Susie has a small child who is often sick. Each time the child is sick, Susie calls into work saying her child is sick and she will not be able to work that day. In doing so, she creates problems for the patients and employees, as everyone scrambles to cover her workload. Although Susie is well liked by both patients and colleagues, the behavior is infuriating and affects the smooth running of the clinic. In this situation, the business owner may choose to terminate this employee, regardless of her stellar contribution while at work. This termination is focused on the concept of care for the greater good. In other words, a good decision for the patients, employees, and the company will be made. When these kinds of decisions are made, they will sometimes reflect poorly on the manager or owner. However, this ethical theory tells us that *only the results are important* and that tough or bad people can achieve good things.

Principled Ethics

The third ethical theory or school of thought is principled ethics. Principled ethics asserts that each person should understand, *in each situation within reason,* what would be the right thing to do and what would be the wrong thing to do. In this principle, the difference between right and wrong leads to actions that are *applied evenly* across each person and each behavior. Let us take the following illustration: your patient has a facial, Botox®, and a dermal filler on the same day. As she moves from the clinician after her facial to the nurse injector, one of her charge tickets is misplaced and it is not caught at the front as she is checking out. She is not charged for the facial, and she does not say a word. The error is caught at the end of the day, and the following day, the manager calls to discuss the problem. The patient tells you that she paid all that was asked of her, and she considers the bill paid in full. In other words, a deal is a deal. If ethical principles were applied evenly and by everyone in a reasonable fashion, the patient would have spoken up on checkout, but she did not; furthermore, she considers the transaction closed once she left your facility.

As we evaluate the topic of ethics, exploring what the concept means for you is important, understanding that three theories of interpretation exist, each of which overlaps in most situations. Whether you are renting a booth or working in a physician's office, situations will come up regularly, and you will need to sort them out and act on them appropriately. Understanding each of these theories and factoring in your personal philosophies will assist you in making every decision.

■ PROFESSIONAL ETHICS

As we have discussed, the two types of ethical codes are personal ethics and professional ethics. These codes too may overlap, just as the ethical theories we have discussed. Nevertheless, each individual document is important. Individually, a code of ethics is a personal document that discusses how you will live your life and what will be your priorities in daily decision making. This document will influence not only you as an individual, but also persons with whom you come into contact, personally and professionally. On the other hand, professional ethics are the guidelines set forth to ensure that each patient or client who comes through your doors are treated with dignity and respect while you maintain a superior clinical treatment. Professional ethics are decided on a larger platform rather than the individual. Professional ethics affect not only the business owner, but also the employees and the clients of the business. Some professional ethics are decided by governmental agencies, called **regulations**, which are mandatory and must be followed at the risk of serious legal consequences. An example of this concept might be the Health Insurance Portability and Accountability Act regulations we face in the medical office. Other guidelines are determined by professional organizations to which we belong or by the spa or clinic that employs you.

regulations
An authoritative rule dealing with details or procedure.

professional code of ethics
The morals held in common by a group of professionals.

Professional Code of Ethics

A **professional code of ethics** should be public and well known to all in our profession, as well as our clients. If we are to be considered a member of trained service professionals (sometimes referred to as allied health professionals) as our counterparts in nursing, social work, nutrition, or other areas are, we should extend ourselves to the highest level, and this includes professional ethics. Therefore exactly what does a code of ethics need to include? "It should discuss appropriate and inappropriate behavior, it should promote high standards of patient care, it should be used for self evaluation, it should establish a framework for professional behavior and responsibilities, it should identify us and create an image of occupational maturity."[7]

Given all of the criteria, we recognize that creating a code of ethics is not an easy task. The National Coalition of Esthetic & Related Associations publishes a code of ethics for aesthetic professionals.

National Coalition of Estheticians, Manufacturers/Distributors and Associations

CLIENT RELATIONSHIPS

Estheticians* will serve the best interests of their clients at all times and will provide the highest quality service possible.

Estheticians will maintain client confidentiality and provide clear, honest communication.

Estheticians will provide clients with clear and realistic goals and outcomes and will not make false claims regarding the potential benefits of the techniques rendered or products recommended.

Estheticians will adhere to the scope of practice of their profession and refer clients to the appropriate qualified health practitioner when indicated.

SCOPE OF PRACTICE

Estheticians will offer services only within the scope of practice as defined by the state within which they operate, if required, and in adherence with appropriate federal laws and regulations.

Estheticians will not use any technique procedure for which they have not had adequate training and shall represent their education, training, qualifications, and abilities honestly.

Estheticians will strictly adhere to all usage instructions and guidelines provided by product and equipment manufacturers, provided these guidelines and instructions are within the scope of practice as defined by the state, if required.

PROFESSIONALISM

Estheticians will commit themselves to ongoing education and provide clients and the public with the most accurate information possible.

Estheticians will dress in attire consistent with professional practice and adhere to the code of conduct of their governing board.

*For the purpose of the NCEA code of ethics, use of the term *esthetician* applies to all licensed skin-care professionals as defined by state law.

Reprinted with permission from the NCEA.

A clinic or spa can use this code as a foundation to customize a document for the facility. Creating a code of professional ethics in your workplace is imperative. This document guides our behavior, promotes high standards, and discusses self-evaluation. The code should also discuss professional maturity and create responsibility.

For a code of ethics to be meaningful, it should be developed by the group that is going to *use* the document. The task may appear overwhelming given that the subject matter can be broad and diverse, especially if the group that is writing the code of ethics is large. The focus of the code is based on moral principles. The process should begin by asking certain questions such as, "Why a code of ethics?" "What is the purpose of our organization?" "What is the purpose of the code?" For the code to be useful, it must reflect the qualities of the group. This point can be difficult because each person within the group has different qualities and moral viewpoints. However, finding a place of compromise is a must if the document is to be useful. The code of ethics must be broad enough to take into consideration the number of people using it but specific enough to direct behavior. Therefore, if the code fails to provide substantive guidance for the organization, it creates confusion. As for the skin-care industry at large and your business specifically, a few tips can be offered (Table 3–2).

Belonging to a professional organization can be educational and a great place to network; but finding a good fit is important. The physician with whom you are working usually belongs to a professional organization. If associations for ancillary staff can be located, consider these organizations first.

"A code of ethics is a means of uniquely expressing a group's collective commitment to a specific set of standards of conduct while offering guidance in how to best follow those codes."[8]

Table 3–2   Writing a Professional Code of Ethics

Component	Considerations
Preamble	What is the purpose of the organization?
Statement of intent	What is the purpose of the code itself?
Fundamental principles	What population is affected by your organization? What is your organization's area of expertise?
Fundamental rules	What unethical situations does your organization want to prevent? What are the likely problem situations in which unethical solutions might arise?
Guidelines for the fundamental principles and fundamental rules	How can these unethical situations be prevented? How can you prevent conflicting principles?

Ethical Dilemmas for Clinicians

Each day that the clinician checks in for work, the potential exists for ethical conflict between the clinician and patients, between the clinician and colleagues, or between the clinician and him or herself. Ethical dilemmas will present themselves in the strangest ways and tug at your soul (Table 3–3).

Take, for example, the woman in your chair with a black eye and bruises on her face. When first questioned, she tells you that she ran into the car door. However, on further discussion, she finally admits to being abused by her husband. She asks you to keep the secret. What do you do? The husband is obviously breaking the law by beating his wife. She wants to leave him, but she is afraid of him. What do you do? This dilemma not only considers the concepts of keeping a secret, but is also complicated by the issues of law. What if he kills her and you knew about the situation?

What about the clinician who is falsifying her time card? You do not want to be a tattletale because she is a single mom and needs the job. However, you struggle. You may wonder what the other employees would think of you for reporting the fraud. In reality, falsifying the time

Table 3–3   Possible Ethical Dilemmas

Ethical Dilemma	Possible Considerations
Keeping a patient's secret	Consider the legal and safety issues.
Knowledge of a dishonest employee	Consider your reputation in the company knowing this information and the "right versus wrong" of stealing.
Patient who complains of treatments by another clinician in your facility	Consider the *greater good* for the company, the patient, and your reputation.
Patient who complains of rudeness of the front desk and telephone staff	Consider the *greater good* for the company, the patient, and your reputation.
Incomplete training	Consider the possibilities of your aptitude and the usual training process versus the right and wrong of the situation.
Patient who is unhappy with a treatment	Consider talking with the patient, and your manager.

card is stealing from the company. What should you do? What would you do?

These kinds of ethical decisions are those that confront the clinicians every day. Sometimes, no decision is a decision. How do you decide what to do? Each time we come to an ethical crossroad, we must collect the facts. Do you perceive the situation from an unbiased rationale, or are external factors involved that may be clouding your judgment? Does it fall into just one ethical theory, or does the situation cross the boundaries of all three theories? Does anyone else see the situation the way you see it? What will be the consequences if nothing is done? What will be the consequences if you do something? We know that all behavior has a consequence, but will you choose the ethical behavior?

Your Moral Compass

A moral compass is an internal monitor that guides and directs you to appropriate behavior that includes justice, virtue, and honesty. By and large, much of the ethical behavior we have been discussing is a product of your upbringing. Morality can be viewed as being on a bell curve. On one extreme, an individual may be considered judgmental or self-righteous if they were brought up by inflexible parents with rigid notions of what is wrong based on prejudice or outdated morality. If, on the other extreme, one of your parents was a thief, your moral code may not be what it should be. In the middle, and the majority, individuals who are reared in a solid family with a parent or parents who believed in them and who let them develop their own morality within the confines of practical judgment, confidence, and conviction will be better prepared to let their moral compass guide them in the right direction. This last instance is how individuals develop a moral compass, by having a strong moral guide when they were young. Your upbringing helps you consider ethical dilemmas and evaluate how to handle them. In families that have solid beliefs in what is *right and wrong,* the dilemma may be solved by open discussions, helping you to find the way. Individuals who are on the extremes can still be guided into thoughtful decision making; however, a more conscientious effort of evaluating the circumstances is more necessary for them. As an adult, you are sensitive to this behavior, and you may want to talk about the options of a situation with friends or spouse. This behavior is underlined with a caring personality and tendencies of compassion, empathy, and sympathy. All of these qualities are common in those of us who seek work in this field.

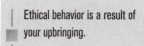
Ethical behavior is a result of your upbringing.

Good Workers

In our capitalist society, we tend to define a good worker in terms of the Protestant work ethic (PWE). In *Confessions of a Workaholic*, Wayne E. Oats summarizes the PWE by stating, "a universal taboo is placed on idleness, and industriousness is considered a religious ideal; waste is a vice, and frugality a virtue; complacency and failure are outlawed, and ambition and success are taken as sure signs of God's favour."[9] According to the PWE, a good worker is closer to divinity, and a lazy worker is closer to the devil. This perspective assumes that all of the productive activities of the good worker are ethical in their nature. Realistically, though, is a good worker ethical? That question is difficult to answer. Although the concepts surely overlap, a separation exists between the two that explains the prevalence of unethical behavior within the highest ranks in some organizations. What, then, defines a good worker? Is a good worker the person who shows up every day and does the job and keeps his or her nose clean? Maybe, but more importantly, being a good worker involves the concept of doing the job in an expert fashion and taking responsibility for that job. These attributes are those that everyone wants in an employee, as a patient, and as a friend. The ideas of being an expert, taking responsibility, and being honest cannot be denied as qualities of a good worker. To have a fair assessment of what characteristics are representative of a good worker, one needs to weave the characteristics of an ethical worker with those of a good worker.

Intrinsic and Extrinsic Satisfaction

In *The Prince*, by Machiavelli, a pragmatic discussion develops that has multiple interpretations. Tweezing out the most compelling components, some people believe what the text says: "If you are going to make a difference in the world, it has to be a difference in the world we live in, not in a theoretic world we would like to live in."[10] Furthermore, "If you're going to make progress in the world you've got to have clear sense, a realistic sense, an unsentimental sense, of how things really work: the mixed motives that compel some people and the high motives that compel others, and the low motives that unfortunately captivate other people."[11] According to Harvard Business School professor Joseph L. Badaracco, this interpretation is the most interesting given by his business school students.

What does this concept mean to you? View and evaluate your world, make it a realistic evaluation. Work within the world as you see it, not as you want it to be. Be pragmatic about your analysis. Understand all the motives of the people with whom you work. Having a complete understanding of the members of your team, the motives of their individual and collective motives, and the goals of your team enables you to make a noticeable contribution to the team. Although this process is difficult and takes time and consideration, when combined with the technical skills, you will become an indispensable member of any teams with which you have membership.

In the working world, the ideas of intrinsic and extrinsic satisfaction can be found with the job. Intrinsic satisfaction involves the idea of doing a great job, better than any one else; it pleases you and makes you proud. The concept of extrinsic satisfaction involves the money you make, the benefits you have, and the recognition you garner.

Intrinsic satisfaction is often the most sustaining and rewarding; however, it is the hardest to achieve because it is all about your inner abilities: your self-esteem and your self-confidence. Your ability to *pat yourself on the back* is especially important because you will sometimes need to do so. The ability to be *proud of yourself* creates inner satisfaction.

Extrinsic satisfaction is full of the concepts you are usually considering but, in reality, will only partially create satisfaction or happiness. The obvious concepts of money and benefits are subjects of constant discussion within the workplace. However, in reality, is money the source of your complete professional happiness? Obviously, being treated fairly is important, but "golden handcuffs" certainly do not create happiness, in fact, quite the opposite. The goal is to ensure that you are fairly treated and garner the kudos of your colleagues and superiors (Table 3–4).

Higher Standard of Professionalism

When we work in the medical office, more is expected of us by both the patient and the physician. We are expected to adhere to a higher level of professionalism and customer service than is familiar to us in the spa setting. Because of the advanced procedures that are performed, and the

Table 3–4   Work Satisfaction Qualities

Intrinsic Satisfaction Qualities	Extrinsic Satisfaction Qualities
Rewards from your inner qualities	Rewards from outside sources
Intact self-esteem	Money
High self-confidence	Recognized as a leader or the "best"
Ability to "pat yourself on the back"	Needs others to "pat you on the back"

skill sets that are required, the clinician must exhibit a level of decorum, whether performing a procedure or not. You must train yourself to refrain from laughing, joking, and loud behavior. Patients may think you are talking or laughing about them. Additionally, that kind of *party* atmosphere does not reflect positively on our image or our profession. In fact, unprofessional behavior can negatively reflect on you in the eyes of the patient. Your ethical conduct should be present in your contact with patients, their charts or records, and your communication with others about the patient. The information you must pass along about the patient to colleagues or others involved in their care should be complete but comply with the Health Insurance Portability and Accountability Act (HIPAA) regulations (see later discussion on page 47). The patient list of the medical spa belongs to the physician, and according to the laws of HIPAA, the information should never leave the medical office.

Matching Ethics in the Workplace

As you finish your resume and begin your search for a new position, an important step is to evaluate your ethics against those of the companies you interview. Our business environment is competitive, and you must understand the rules of the game; this is the first litmus test for your ethics. Ask the interviewer if the company has a defined set of ethical guidelines. Consider each one, and decide if they are compatible with your own beliefs. If, in the end, the patient and honest business dealings are not the primary ethical considerations, you may want to consider other options.

Ethics in the Salon and Spa

Business ethics and professional principles should not differ from one another. However, the difference exists between telling the truth and doing the right thing. The right thing is far more involved than a simple "yes" or "no" of the truth.

Americans are a litigious people. Lawsuits are filed at the drop of a hat. Therefore the aesthetician must bear in mind that he or she can be the focus of a lawsuit simply by providing service. So how can the aesthetician perform the daily functions of the job and be protected each day?

Take, for example, the client who has a facial and develops a rash from the standard products used in a facial. Did she tell you she was allergic to anything before the facial? Once developing the rash, she insists on a refund. What is the right course of action? You did the work and provided the service. The client did not disclose any allergy before or after the service. What is the best long-term decision for the aesthetician and the medical spa? Each person will have the answer that fits for them, but let us consider some potential debate points. First, did the clinician do anything wrong? Certainly not. Did the patient sign a waiver before treatment? Assuming that everything was done as required, the patient's money should not be refunded. On the other hand, is that the right decision? Generally, a payoff or a refund implies an admission of guilt. Is it doing the right thing to admit to a mistake and assume guilt when you do not believe that you are in the wrong? What does *right* involve? How would you feel if you were this patient? Would you want the spa to acknowledge your hardship? Can an ethical compromise be reached?

These are the kinds of situations and questions that the clinician must be capable of addressing. Dilemmas such as these should pass the sleep test.[12] The sleep test is defined as *what keeps you awake at night.* Did you make the right decision that allows a peaceful sleep?

Ethics in the Medical Spa

The foundation of the medical relationship is built on trust, caring, compassion, and truth. The relationship is sustained by confidentiality, accuracy in treatment, and putting the patient's welfare at the peak. The role of the clinician in the medical spa is different than that of the clinician in the luxury spa. Behavior in a medical spa is more clearly dictated by medical rules and regulations than in the day-to-day business arena. Although the medical environment may hold its practitioners to a higher standard, the reality is that the standards are still based in ethics, the right versus wrong paradigm. It is safe to say that in the medical spa, every action and treatment must intentionally attempt to fulfill the mutual goals of the clinician and the patient. Simplifying the right versus wrong paradigm should take us back to simple concepts such as ethics of duties or ethics of consequences,[13] which are so powerful in the medical world. Although some of us may have the intuition of knowing the right answer, in reality, many problems in the medical spa can be complex and without a correct answer. Additionally, beauty is in the eye of the beholder. To this effect, consider what is driving the treatment: the patient or the protocol of the clinic. Therefore clarity in consultation and in treatment instructions often directs the end result.

■ WHERE TO FIND ETHICAL GUIDANCE

Being a good worker and an ethical worker is a difficult and active process. When done in solitude, the possibility exists that your own morality may not be consistent with the ethical practices suited for the aesthetics industry. Whether you believe this to be personally relevant, everyone considering a career in aesthetics should know where he or she can seek out ethical guidance. Several resources can help you fine tune your ethical responsibilities, as well as enhance the more technical aspects of your job performance.

Regulatory Agencies

The agencies that regulate the spas are not federalized but implemented on a state-by-state basis. Therefore you must check with the licensing agency in your state to determine any specific requirements that relate to your job, aside from general licensure. For example, you might need a certificate indicating that you have completed a course on microdermabrasion to perform the treatment.

Professional Organizations

Our industry is fractured. Many organizations are trying to accomplish lofty goals for our industry only to be in conflict with another organization with the same goals. Supporting organizations that have our best interests in mind and that work toward goals to create uniform educational requirements will be important over the coming years for us. The most progressive organization is the NCEA, which is an umbrella association for the many small organizations in the marketplace. Check with NCEA to find out if a professional organization exists that meets your individual needs. Meanwhile, if you work for a plastic surgeon, check

HIPAA Regulates the Medical Office

When working in a medical office, the clinician must understand all of the laws and regulations that affect the practice. Among these rules and laws is the HIPAA. Passed by Congress in 1996 and signed into law in January of 1997, the purpose of this Act is to protect the privacy of patients' health information. Uniform standards are now implemented across the nation that identify how health information changes hands. Health information is protected by stringent rules that apply to information in the chart, on the computer or fax, and by spoken word. Seven categories of the law are of concern to our industry. These categories include access to medical records, notice of privacy practices, limits on use of personal medical information, prohibition on marketing, stronger state law, confidential communications, and complaints.[14]

into the Society of Plastic Surgical Skin Care Specialists, and if you work for a dermatologist, check into the Society of Dermatology Skin Care Specialists.

Find a Role Model

The landscape of the medical spa can be littered with landmines for the clinician. Situations that are seen and evaluated can often be avoided; however, in some instances, the eyes of a colleague or role model will help the clinician grow and become a valuable member of the team.

One of the best strategies for a new clinician or a clinician striving to improve him or herself is to find a role model. This process will help you identify and try out different professional *personalities*. What do we mean by this statement? Well, you have a personal identity, the part of you that is shared with family and loved ones. However, in the business world, you have a different *you*. The *business world you* often needs development and attention to detail. A role model or mentor can help you reach this goal. A difference exists between learning factual knowledge and refining the professional personality to use these skills. Many times, a single role model is not enough. Only parts of the style are compatible, or single components of the personality are a match. Therefore developing relationships with multiple role models is important to achieve a meaningful result. We should be realistic: one person cannot bring all of the details into focus for you (Table 3–5).

Role Model Strategies

Role models are important for the beginning clinician. A role model to the clinician is someone he or she would want to "be like" and develop a strategy to get to that end point. Role models are important for clinicians who are striving to create a growth career, a place where they will improve and grow. This task simply cannot be done alone and requires the help of a role model.

Table 3–5 Benefits of a Role Model

Someone against whom to model professional behavior
Sorts out the *pains* of professional growth
Gives direction, ideas, and suggestions for growth
Is a resource and *sounding board*

Your role model need not even know you are modeling after him or her. The main thing is that you are taking the positive behaviors and creating a professional persona that is superior to your current persona.

Two role model strategies are defined as imitation strategies and true-to-self strategies.[15] Imitation role modeling is simply that: an imitation. In the true-to-self model, the individual takes key components from the role model and implements them into his or her own behavior, creating a strategy that allows him or her to *own* the changes.

Imitation role modeling requires the identification of a senior person, one with varied experience. In identifying such a person, the clinician is able to compare his or her skills against those of the role model in both clinical skills and communication skills. In doing so, the clinician should be able to notice the variables that he or she would like to *try out* and experiment with to acquire a more professional and skilled persona. This process is trial and error, as compared with factual learning. In factual learning, the clinician is given a set of facts to be learned or memorized. Imitation role modeling is much more esoteric: identifying actions and deeds of another and then perfecting them through trial and error.

True-to-self role modeling involves the participant collecting information from the role model and then incorporating it into behaviors that will work for him or her. The idea is really to be yourself,[16] using ideas, concepts, and routines that work for you. This method creates an authenticity that is often more comfortable for the participant and certainly easier to use. However, this process is harder to implement and requires more work and recognition of self. Limitations may be encountered because the ideas or concepts simply do not fit into the natural behaviors of the participant.

> Your professional identity is who you are in a professional role; it is a unique identity that is different than who you are at home or with friends.

Your Professional Identity

"Your professional identity is defined as the relatively stable and enduring collection of attributes, beliefs, values, motives and experiences which people define themselves in a professional role (Schein, 1978)."[17] In other words, professional identity is what you are when you are in your professional role. Clinicians who work hard to develop a unique professional identity, one with which patients can be comfortable, are the most successful clinicians. It requires, as you have read, a role model who allows experimentation and strategies that foster professional growth and development. Practicing is an essential component of developing a unique professional identity. Becoming the professional you want to be will take time. Sometimes, you will be clumsy and awkward; other times, you will feel comfortable and easy. Remember the comfortable and easy times; this is the professional identity that will suit you best.

■ PATIENT RIGHTS

Achieving an optimal outcome requires a certain amount of effort and participation on the parts of both the clinician and the patient. Aside from the more clinical aspects of treatment, such as the consultation or the care plan, some of the more esoteric, albeit commonsense, regulations need to be followed.

For clinicians who are new to the medical field, patients have rights —true rights—outlined by law. In 1996 President Clinton appointed a commission to address many health care issues in our nation. Included was the concept that has become known as *consumer rights and responsibilities*. In 1998 the commission issued its report, and the document now known as the Consumer Bill of Rights and Responsibilities was introduced.

As patients and consumers, we take these rights seriously; and as care givers, we should also seriously consider the rights of patients. The Consumer Bill of Rights takes into consideration the following topics: informed disclosure, choice of provider and plans, access to emergency services, participation in treatment decisions, respect and nondiscrimination, confidentiality of health information, complaints and appeals, and fees.[18] Obviously, not all of these topics are applicable or appropriate for the medical spa or day spa. However, the clinician should still be aware of the entire document and the individual components. Therefore we will discuss each of the individual components and how they might relate to the spa industry.

> The Consumer Bill of Rights and Responsibilities was introduced in 1998.

> The Consumer Bill of Rights and Responsibilities has many sections. Some sections are applicable to the medical spa, and some are not. The clinician should be familiar with the document and which components are important to him or her and the job he or she does each day.

Informed Disclosure

Informed disclosure is the first consumer right that is discussed in the bill. Disclosure obviously means to disclose or to be open about a subject. However, informed disclosure means that the patient has the right to *understand* his or her health care. Therefore the disclosure goes beyond the process of being open and is burdened by understandable information. The document goes further to say that the patient has the right to understand not only the information about their health condition, but also about the health care professionals and facility. If the patient does not speak the language spoken in the clinic, the language barrier must be addressed so that the patient can receive the necessary information. What does this concept mean for the medical spa? First, it means that the patient must always be told what procedure is being done for him or her. Even if the procedure is done repeatedly, the clinician must go through the steps and make sure the patient understands the process. Informed disclosure also means that the clinician should wear a nametag for identification. The nametag should contain both the first and the last name, as well as the credentials, of the clinician. Finally, the clinician is obligated to ensure that the patient understands the facility: its purpose and layout.

Choice of Providers and Plans

Choice of providers and plans means that the patient has the right to choose health care providers within their insurance plan. It also means that the patient has the right to have a choice about their insurance plans. Obviously, the medical spa may be an arm's reach from this concept. Nearly all, if not all, of the treatments provided by the medical spa are fee for service; in other words, the insurance company will not cover the treatment. However, if the medical spa is located in a dermatology office, for example, the clinician may be asked questions about insurance or be involved in the insurance process, depending on his or her job description.

Access to Emergency Services

Access to emergency services allows the patient to seek services in the emergency facilities of a hospital or clinic without preauthorization. Once again, rarely is the clinician involved in this situation. However, on rare occasions, a peel or treatment may cause a patient undue pain, and your physician may recommend that the patient seek treatment at the local emergency room. This circumstance, however, would be unusual. Therefore being faced with implementing this patient right would be unusual for the clinician.

Participation in Treatment

Participation in treatment decisions is a consumer right and one that the clinician will often find him or herself implementing. This component means that the patient has the right not only to understand about the treatment, but also to make decisions about the treatment. To comply with this consumer right, the clinician will be providing a lot of education for the patient. The patient will need to understand what the treatment options are and which treatment will work best for the problem at hand. Therefore the clinician should have predictable treatment descriptions, before and after photographs, and experiential recommendations to comply with this component of the document.

Respect and Nondiscrimination

Respect and nondiscrimination is also a consumer right. Many of the rights found in this document are important, but, inarguably, respect and nondiscrimination must be at the top of the list. Each patient should be treated with respect, throughout the treatment process and without discrimination.

Confidentiality

Confidentiality of health information means that all patients can expect their health care information to be kept confidential. As we all now know, this point has been taken further and developed into the concept called HIPAA. All patients have the right to be assured that their information is being kept confidential and safe. Patients also have the right to review their medical records and request that amendments be made if inaccuracies exist.

Complaints and Appeals

Complaints and appeals are also a consumer right. This component involves a process of resolving discrepancies. These discrepancies can include items as minimal as waiting times and hours of operation to more significant aspects such as professional conduct. The patient has a right to a fair and speedy review process of any complaint. Obviously, we address these kinds of problems daily in the medical spa as a process of customer service.

> Abiding by patient rights gives the clinician a guideline for professional behavior.

Fees

Finally, in the medical spa, the patient has the right to understand the charges to be billed before the service begins. In the spa setting, this right means that you cannot push any products and services that patients do not want or products or services they consider superfluous. As a clinician, your responsibility will be to know which products are critical to the success of the treatment and which ones can be optional.

▪ PATIENT RESPONSIBILITIES

A good relationship always has two sides: a give and take. Although the professional has many responsibilities in the patient–medical professional relationship, the patient also has responsibilities. Therefore for what exactly might the patient be responsible in this relationship? In fact, a significant list of responsibilities exists for the patient; let us take a look.

Accurate Information

First, the patient must provide accurate and complete information to the clinic, including name, age, past illness (and associated care), medications (including herbal medicines), and any other vital information. Additionally, the patient should provide accurate contact information: address, telephone numbers, social security number, insurance information, and employer information. Another responsibility of patients is to ask questions that are pertinent to their health and get answers to things they do not understand.

Pain Tolerance

The patient should also communicate to the clinician about pain tolerance. This information helps the clinician make the patient more comfortable during procedures such as Botox® or dermal fillers.

Abide by Rules

Finally, abiding by the clinic's rules is important for the patient. If your clinic has a no-smoking policy (which most do), the patient should respect this rule. Other regulations may include the consideration of other patients (e.g., no children, no cell phones, no loud talking).

> Clear and precise communication is the ultimate goal of the paradigm defined in the Consumer Bill of Rights and Responsibilities.

TOP TEN TIPS TO TAKE TO THE CLINIC

1. We should never leave our ethics at the business door; they should be used daily. In other words, be true to yourself.
2. The discussion of ethics is not a simple issue of right and wrong.
3. Your patient may view ethical behavior that is different from your view and your employer.
4. No difference should exist between workplace ethics and personal ethics.
5. Large cities, large businesses, and expanded exposures to people and situations challenge our ethics.
6. Patient rights are important to understand and apply, when appropriate, in your practice.
7. Patients have the responsibility of being honest and complete in the information they disclose.
8. The information that patients disclose can make a difference in the treatment or program that is selected for them.
9. Abiding by the Consumer Bill of Rights and Responsibilities gives the clinician a guideline for professional behavior.
10. Clear communication is the goal of the Consumer Bill of Rights and Responsibilities.

CHAPTER REVIEW QUESTIONS

1. What are ethics?
2. What types of ethical situations might occur in the medical spa?
3. How might you handle an unethical situation?
4. How do you achieve intrinsic and extrinsic work satisfaction?
5. What are the Consumer Bill of Rights and Responsibilities?
6. What is spa etiquette?
7. How does the Consumer Bill of Rights and Responsibilities differ from spa etiquette?
8. How do these concepts help us develop a relationship with our patients or clients?

BIBLIOGRAPHY

Badaracco, J. L. Jr. (1997, March). *Defining moments: When managers must choose between right and wrong. Boston: HBS Press.*

Barad, R. (2004). *Laser skin resurfacing,* [Online]. Available: www.laserexpert.com

Bernard, R. W., Beran, S. J., & Rusin, L. (2000, October). Microdermabrasion in clinical practice. *Journal of Clinical Plastic Surgery,* 27(4), 571–577.

Brennan, H. G. (2001, April). Skin care in my practice: The spectrum concept. *North American Journal of Facial and Plastic Surgery,* 9(3), 383–394.

Briket, W. P. (2000, July). *Ethical codes in action* [Online]. Available: www.ifac.org

Brody, H. J., Geronemus, R. G., & Faris, P. K. (2003, April). Beauty versus medicine: The non-physician practice of dermatologic surgery. *Journal of Dermatologic Surgery,* 29(4), 319–324.

Callen, J. P., Paller, A. S., Greer, K. E., & Swinyer, L. J. (2000). *Color atlas of dermatology* (2nd ed.). Philadelphia: W. B. Saunders.

D' Angelo, J., Dean, P., Dietz, S., Hinds, C., Lees, M., Miller, E., et al. (2003). *Milady's standard: Comprehensive training for estheticians.* Clifton Park, NY: Thomson Delmar Learning.

Deitz, S. (2004). *Milady's the clinical esthetician.* Clifton Park, NY: Thomson Delmar Learning.

Dobrin, A. (2002). *Ethics for everyone.* New York: Wiley and Sons.

Freeman, S. (2001, May). Microdermabrasion. *North American Journal of Facial and Plastic Surgery,* 9(2), 257–266.

Gerson, J. (2004). *Milady's standard: Fundamentals for estheticians* (9th ed.). Clifton Park, NY: Thomson Delmar Learning.

Goldberg, G. (2004, January 15). *Microdermabrasion* [Online]. Available: www.pimaderm.com

Guttman, C. (2002, August). Histologic studies: Microdermabrasion not just superficial. *Cosmetic Surgery Times* [Online]. Available: http://www.pimaderm.com

Heskett, J. (2003, June 30). *Summing up: What can aspiring leaders be taught?* [Online]. Available: http://www.hbsworkingknowledge.hbs.edu

Hinds, A. (2003, August 30). *Not convinced yet? Aestheticians turn the tide, washing in new oppoprtunities* [Online]. Available: www.cosmeticsurgerytimes.com

Koch, R. J., Hanasono, N. M. (2001, August). Microdermabrasion. *North American Journal of Facial and Plastic Surgery, 9*(3), 377–382.

Lavington, C., Losee, S. (2001). *You've only got three seconds.* New York: Broadway Books.

Lee, W. R., Shen, S. C., Kuo-Hsien, W., Hu, C. H., & Fang, J. Y. (2003, November). Lasers and microdermabrasion enhance and control topical delivery of vitamin C. *Journal of Investigative Dermatology, 121*(5), 1118–1125.

Lloyd, J. R. (2002, August). The use of microdrermabrasion for acne: A pilot study. *Journal of Dermatologic Surgery, 27*(4), 329–331.

MacDonald, C. (2004, March). *Guidance for writing a code of ethics* [Online]. Available: www.ethics.web.ca

Oslon, A. (2004, March). *Authoring a code: Observations on process and organization* [Online]. Available: www.iit.edu

Palmer, G. D. (2001, October). Regarding the study on microdermabrasion on acne. *Journal of Dermatological Surgery, 27*(10), 914.

Pilla, L. (2002, October). *Medical spas: Where medicine and luxury meet in the middle* [Online]. Available: www.skinandaging.com

Poulos, S. (2004, March). *Erbium laser skin resurfacing* [Online]. Available: www.poulosmd.com

Prague Aesthetic Surgery. (2004, March). *CO_2 laser & erbium laser: Skin smoothing & non-invasive facial rejuvination* [Online]. Available: www.aesthetia.com

Rath, T., & Clifton, D. (2004). *How full is your bucket?* New York: Gallup.

Rubin, M. (1995). *Manual of chemical peels: Superficial and medium depth.* Philadelphia: Lippincott, Williams & Wilkins.

Shim, E. K., Barnette, D., Hughes, K., & Greenway, H. G. (2001, June). Microdermabrasion: A clinical and histopathic study. *Journal of Dermatologic Surgery, 27*(6) 524–530.

Sodroski, A. (2003, December). *Something like a rich widow: Spartacus and the Protestant work ethic* [Online] Available: www.pages. emerson.edu

United States Department of Health and Human Services. (2004, March 9). *Fact sheet* [Online]. Available: www.hhs.gov

Merriam-Webster's Collegiate Dictionary, (1992). New York: Random House.

Von Baeyer, C. (2004). *What's workplace ethics?* [Online] www. workplaceethics.ca

Whitaker, E. (2003, December 2). *Microdermabrasion,* [Online]. Available: www.emedicine.com

CHAPTER REFERENCES

1. Badaracco, Jr., J. L. (1997). *Defining moments* Boston: Harvard Business School Press.
2. Von Baeyer, C. (2004). *What's workplace ethics?* [On line] Available: http://www.workplaceethics.ca
3. *Merriam-Webster's Collegiate Dictionary.* (1992). New York: Random House.
4. Dobrin, A. (2002). *Ethics for everyone, how to increase your moral intelligence.* New York: John Wiley & Sons.
5. Dobrin, A. (2002). *Ethics for everyone, how to increase your moral intelligence.* New York: John Wiley & Sons.
6. Dobrin, A. (2002). *Ethics for everyone, how to increase your moral intelligence.* New York: John Wiley & Sons.
7. MacDonald, C. (2004, March 9). *Why have a code of ethics?* [Online] Available: http://www.ethicsweb.ca
8. Oslon, A. (2004, March 11). *Authoring a code: Observations on process and organization* [Online] Available: http://www.iit.edu
9. Sodroski, A. (2003, December). *Something like a rich widow: Spartacus and the Protestant work ethic* [Online]. Available: http://pages. emerson.edu
10. Heskett, J. (2003, June 30). *Summing up: What can aspiring leaders be taught?* [Online]. Available: http://www.hbsworkingknowledge.hbs.edu
11. Badaracco, Jr., J. L. (1997). *Defining moments* Boston Harvard Business School Press.
12. Badaracco, Jr., J. L. (1997). *Defining moments.* Boston: Harvard Business School Press.
13. Badaracco, Jr., J. L. (1997). *Defining moments.* Boston: Harvard Business School Press.

14. United States Department of Health and Human Services. (2004, March 9). *Fact sheet* [Online] Available: http://www.hhs.gov

15. Heskett, J. (2003, June 30). *Summing up: What can aspiring leaders be taught?* [Online] Available: http://www.hbsworkingknowledge.hbs.edu

16. Heskett, J. (2003, June 30). *Summing up: What can aspiring leaders be taught?* [Online] Available: http://www.hbsworkingknowledge.hbs.edu

17. Heskett, J. (2003, June 30). *Summing up: What can aspiring leaders be taught?* [Online] Available: http://www.hbsworkingknowledge.hbs.edu

18. United States Department of Health and Human Services. (2004, March 9). *Fact sheet* [Online] Available: http://www.hhs.gov

Consultations

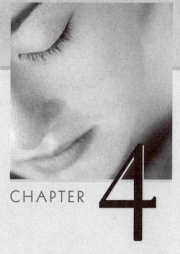

CHAPTER 4

KEY TERMS

body dysmorphic
  disorder
Botox®
consultation
Cosmoderm® and
  Cosmoplast®

Fitzpatrick skin typing
  worksheet
health history sheet
Help Us Understand You
  sheet
Hylaform®

image business
impressions
patient information sheet
perception
Restylane®
skin history sheet

LEARNING OBJECTIVES

After completing this chapter you should be able to:

1. Discuss the purpose of the consultation.
2. Define how consultations are used in the care of patients.
3. Discuss the importance of telephone consultations.
4. Discuss customer service and the consultative process.

INTRODUCTION

In earlier chapters, we examined some of the broader theories of sociology and communication that will play a role in your professional success. From these theories, we can compound our knowledge a little more by examining some of the day-to-day situations during which you will employ the aforementioned concepts, thus increasing the likelihood of achieving a consistent, attainable, and positive outcome for the client and yourself.

Membership in the medical and allied medical fields can be complicated in its multifactorial and multifunctional capacities. Knowing which skills to employ at what moment or "in synch" with other skills you have will require you to embark in a delicate dance between form and function with the appearance of ease and professionalism. Some schools of thought say a person will not remember information until the concept is repeated eight times.[1] Hence this seemingly difficult tasking is made easier with time and experience. However, as mentioned already, having the educational foundation will give you the leg up needed before entering the clinical environment.

Having the knowledge is only one aspect of success in the aesthetics industry. Your successes are often driven by the **impressions** people have of you and the aesthetic industry. We are in an **image business**. The first impression a new patient will have of your office and your expertise is based, in part, on the cleanliness of the office, the knowledge and friendliness of the staff, and, last but certainly not least, your appearance.

During the **consultation**, a patient's ability to listen and hear your information is affected by how comfortable they feel. This *comfort zone* includes how *medicinal* the room appears (this can be intimidating), the seating arrangement, and your professionalism. Professionalism relates to your appearance, knowledge, and command of the language. Mastering the skills of friendliness, cleanliness, comfort, professionalism, and communication can affect the patient's first and lasting impressions.

Furthermore, the **perception** the patient has of you is one that extends to your physician, your colleagues, and the rest of the staff at the spa. The impression the patient has of you and the facility will determine trust, which is the foundation of any relationship.

impressions

A collection of lasting opinions or judgments of something.

image business

A type of business on which the way the public views the company is based largely on how things look, or how they are perceived, more so than actual performance.

consultation

The initial visit with a professional during which the client and the professional both investigate whether a specific treatment or service is warranted or achievable.

perception

Cognitive awareness or recognition. What the patient thinks of you.

CONSULTATION

The first and arguably the most obvious opportunity to use your skills will be during the consultative process. This is the point at which you will meet the client, listen to his or her complaints, investigate the client's skin-care objectives, decipher the degree to which you can help, devise a care plan, and make the steps necessary to realization of the objectives.

Most importantly, the consultation process is your opportunity to familiarize yourself with the client and, from your inferences, customize each client's clinical experience to suit his or her physical, emotional, and psychologic needs.

Consultation is the term used for the conversation you have with a patient when you are on a *fact-finding* mission. The objective of the consultation is to gather information both objective and subjective that will help ensure that the care of the patient will be goal directed toward a desired treatment result.

Outwardly, the consultative process may appear to be for the client's benefit, but as you will soon see, this process benefits the clinician and the clinic just as much if not to a greater degree. The client will benefit from revised expectations set forth from an individualized care plan. The clinician will benefit from a well-planned and executed treatment. The clinic itself will benefit from a team of personnel who can repeatedly optimize their performance over a period. To achieve as much, the consultative procedures can be initiated in several ways.

Therefore what is the best consultation process? Does only one precise process exist? If it is flexible, how so? All of these questions are important aspects to ensure the consultation process is one that meets the needs and desires of the patient, the clinician, and the clinic. Fundamentally, the needs of the clinician and the clinic cannot be met unless the patient needs are met. How do we ensure that we have done so?

By streamlining the consultative processes, using all available resources, and employing communication and psychologic devices to overturn all stones, the treatments selected will have greater chances for success. First, we will examine some of the procedural aspects of aesthetics that will streamline and organize the consultative procedures.

Consultative Process from an Administrative Perspective

From a clinical point of view, the objective of the consultation is to determine the patient's candidacy for a particular procedure, for example, a glycolic acid peel or microdermabrasion.

As we have discussed, the true mutual objective of the patient and clinician is this: improving the patient's appearance. The patient came to you because he or she has a *need* to look better. You are in your position because, through your education and experience, you can *fulfill* this need.

Consultation Paperwork

The recommended paperwork for the skin-care consultation consists of five documents: the **patient information sheet**, the **health history sheet**, the **skin history sheet**, the **Fitzpatrick skin typing worksheet**, and the **Help Us Understand You sheet**. As you will note, each document has an independent and specific use.

The patient information sheet (PI sheet) is the document that captures all of the social information, e-mail addresses, and referral sources. This sheet contains a wealth of information. It tells us where the client lives, where he or she works (or does not work), if the client is married or has a partner, and what his or her interests are in our business.

The health history sheet covers the patient's health. It will address the current chronic or acute diseases, medications that the client may take, and physicians that the client sees. This information will help the clinician determine whether the patient is a candidate for chemical peeling.

The skin history sheet contains a history of the skin conditions, skin treatments, and the products the patient is currently using. It will also have information such as previous product use and skin sensitivities, if any. You will also want this sheet to show information on services the patient has had and the responses to these services.

The Fitzpatrick skin typing worksheet is a group of collective worksheets that determine the patient's skin type. Given that skin typing is a critical aspect of the consultation process, these worksheets, though completed by the patient, must be reviewed for accuracy by the clinician. The skin type will influence the home-care program, the clinical program, and, finally, the potential result.

The Help Us Understand You sheet is a communication and evaluation tool. The questions on this sheet ask the patient to grade his or her knowledge, communication style, and preferences for skin care. This important tool will help you guide and direct the conversations and teaching in ways to which your patient will be more receptive.

You must understand your patient, the patient's health history, and his or her motivations before making any substantive recommendations in consultation. For you to have a truly complete picture of each individual situation, a complete and easy-to-interpret document will be essential. Furthermore, the process will allow for a simplified transfer of information to your co-workers and specialists who may also be coming in contact with a patient. The patient should complete this documentation before the first visit, and the clinician should review and complete the document during the consultation.

Among the assorted documents that new clients will complete on their first visit will be the *skin history sheet* and the *health history sheet*. Although these two documents sound similar in nature, both will offer you detailed and specific information that represent a critical aspect of your responsibilities. These documents are often completed rather quickly and thoughtlessly. As a professional tending to the medical and aesthetic needs of your client, ensuring that the documents are complete and intelligible is ultimately your responsibility.

The skin history sheet is a detailed questionnaire about the patient's skin. You will want to ask questions in the survey that include the past skin health and current skin health. Some of the specific items you will want to know are past and current tanning habits, including sunburns (as a child and as an adult), skin cancer diagnoses, and locations of skin cancers. Additionally, ask about moles or lesions that concern the patient, including their location. Information regarding past and current acne concerns that includes the medications used (both oral and topical) is vital. You must also be aware of previous skin treatments, x-ray treatments for acne, and psoralen ultraviolet A (PUVA) treatments for psoriasis, as well as the usual spa treatments such as facials and body treatments and any problems associated with these treatments. Finally, you will want to ask about basics such as skin condition (oily, dry, normal, sensitive, combination) and skin type. This document will help you fully understand the patient's overall skin health. It will also give you a clearer history, not just what the clients chooses to tell you verbally.

The skin history sheet can also help you understand the segments of your practice. For example, how many patients do you see who have had a skin cancer? How many patients do you see with acne? How many patients do you see who tan? Some of this information would be valuable to your marketing department and for possible future advertising promotions.

Make sure that the client completely fills out the health history and skin history sheets. These histories represent a great place to start the conversation. "Mrs. Smith, I am going to take a moment and acquaint myself with your history. Please bear with me a moment while I become familiar with your history." Take a moment and look through the information that the patient has provided and ask relevant questions to fill in the areas that are incomplete. An incomplete area usually means the answer to the question is "no," but sometimes it may mean the patient did not want to give the information or unintentionally skipped the question. Do not leave any blanks. Ask the patient to finish filling out the document if an area is incomplete. Be sure you review both the health history and the skin history sheets. Add anything relevant as you go through documents with the client. Make notes on your consultation sheet, not on the documents that the patient filled out. Take this part of the consultation seriously, and make notes that will help you help the patient.

The health history sheet asks detailed health status. This questionnaire delves into the past and current health of your patient. Included on this document are questions regarding allergies, current and past illness, smoking status, pregnancy status, daily medications, and past surgical events. The objective of the health history sheet is to obtain a detailed *snap shot* of the client's health without spending a lot of time. This form should be set up in a check-box format. Although the client may think that some of the health items are irrelevant, the questions may be important in delivering care, and all boxes should be checked "yes" or "no."

Knowing the medications that the patient is taking is an important step in the long-term result, which includes regular medications such as birth control pills or antibiotics such as tetracycline. These medications, as well as others, can affect the pigment of the skin. Another important group of medications are those that make the skin sun sensitive. You will want to be sure to educate your patient about this group of medications.

A history of herpes simplex (cold sores) is critical for the clinician to know because glycolic acid, or any peel for that matter, can stimulate an eruption of a lesion. Microdermabrasion has also been shown to stimulate cold sores in patients who are prone to breakouts. Medications have been developed to control the outbreak of herpes simplex, and these medications should be a required part of the treatment protocol for patients who are susceptible to developing an outbreak (Table 4–1).

Table 4–1   Important Information in Consultative Paperwork

Form	Important Information
Personal information sheet	Referral source, social information
Health history sheet	Illnesses, medications, chronic diseases
Skin history sheet	Product use, previous treatments, current problems
Help Us Understand You sheet	How best to communicate issues of importance to the patient

■ MAXIMIZING YOUR RESOURCES

In the clinical environment, a plentitude of resources will be available. Educational resources that include training, conferences, and continuing education will all be valuable to keep you up to date on all the most current procedures. However, the most valuable resource will be closer to home.

Team Approach to Consultations

The best consultation for the patient is a team consultation. A *team consultation* is a process during which several experts within the clinic provide accurate, complete answers for the patient. Two common consultative processes have been developed. Neither process is particularly organized or efficient for the medical spa, which is quite problematic given that the most important conversation you will have with the patient will be the consultative conversation. However, first, let us review the common approaches to consultations in the medical spa or luxury spa environment.

First, the patient comes for cosmetic surgery reasons and is examined by the physician. The conversation with the physician can be lengthy and sometimes involve an examination; such is the case in breast augmentation or liposuction. When the consultation is complete and all the questions have been answered, the physician may recommend that the patient see the aesthetician. After a lengthy consultation with the physician and a focus on cosmetic surgery, the patient may often be reluctant to proceed to a skin-care consultation at this appointment. The patient may be tired or just focused on the information that the physician discussed. Skin care may be the last thing on the patient's mind. In any event, the patient is then referred to the skin-care department to be examined by the aesthetician. Ideally, the aesthetician should give the patient a skin-care packet and schedule a dedicated appointment for discussion of skin-care matters.

The second common avenue of entry into the practice will be through the skin-care consultation itself. In this scenario, the patient will be *primarily* interested in skin-care problems and is scheduled for consultation with the aesthetician. During this consultation, the patient will be focused on the nonsurgical approaches to a more youthful appearance. Questions about dermal injectables such as **Cosmoderm® and Cosmoplast®**, as well as **Restylane®** and **Hylaform®**, will be of interest to the patient. Additionally, questions about **Botox®** are likely to come up. The clinician must have access to materials and a nurse to answer all of the questions clearly and accurately. The clinician may believe that he or she has adequate training, but the clinician providing

Cosmoderm® and Cosmoplast®
Dermal fillers that are a variation on traditional bovine collagen using human collagen.

Restylane®
A dermal filler using non-animal-based hyaluronic acid.

Hylaform®
A dermal filler using animal-based hyaluronic acid.

Botox®
Trade name for small doses of the botulism toxin (*Clostridium botulinum*) that are injected into the wrinkle-causing muscles. The toxin blocks the release of the chemicals that would otherwise signal the muscle to contract, thus paralyzing the injected muscle.

the treatment will have the most up-to-date information. Therefore, if you have a nurse injector, know where he or she is and if this person is able to step in for an introduction during your conversation. This approach will help the clinic's credibility and the patient's willingness to trust the facility.

If the patient is new to the facility, he or she may have questions about plastic surgery. Although getting the physician into your room for a quick consultation is difficult, the patient coordinator should always be available. The patient coordinator for the plastic surgeon is the employee who is responsible for educating patients, preparing them for surgery, scheduling the surgery, and collecting fees. The patient coordinator obviously has a lot of information at his or her fingertips and is a good resource for the clinician.

Being resourceful and knowledgeable is the responsibility of the aesthetician. Collaborating with colleagues and working with the patient to achieve the best possible outcome will serve the patient and the clinician well.

Reference Materials

Literature is among the most important items to have available. These documents, when they are well done, are the best sales tool you will have. Although developing and printing your own literature is expensive, doing so is the best way to go. Literature exhibits originality, confidence, and a positive image. This literature does not have to be extensive or have multiple-color for that matter; it just needs to explain the procedure and positively reflect on the facility.

A photo album of before and after treatment results is a nice tool for use during a consultation. Whether the results you are discussing are microdermabrasion, Botox®, or cosmetic surgery results, pictures can say a thousand words. Be sure you have an album that allows the patient to see the results that you have achieved and those of your colleagues. Be careful, however, that photographs do not misrepresent to the patient that the same exact results can be achieved for them. This problem is common and difficult; a patient sees a picture and assumes that this result is *normal*. Each person is different and should be treated as such, remembering that the skin is different, the problems are different, and, most importantly, the patient participant can vary, therefore influencing the result. This disclaimer should appear on each page of photographs.

Literature should also be provided that describes the facility, the philosophy of the facility, the employees (this should be a lift-out sheet for easy replacement), the history of the practice, and any other relevant components that would help communicate your brand.

> Do not show photographs to the patient that may misrepresent the exact results that can be achieved for them. Photographs should be used as a teaching tool.

Finally, a price menu should be included in the literature, which should also should be a lift-out sheet that is easy to replace when prices change.

Different Office Consultative Processes

First, put yourself in your patient's shoes. You have heard this old cliché a million times, but really put yourself in the patient's shoes. Sit in your waiting area, listen to the front desk chatter, sit in the treatment chairs, have your photograph taken, and really try to go through the process. What do you like about the process? For example, do you want to fill out paperwork in the waiting area or in a private room? Do you want to change clothes in a locker room, in the treatment room, or in a private dressing area attached to the treatment room? Some of this process will obviously be dictated by the footprint of your facility and your ability to work around the physical space. However, really think it through, and consider the privacy, comfort, and sensibility of the processes you have set up. What do you think warrants a change? These are questions to ask and represent a place to begin making positive change.

Once you have gone through the process yourself and made the necessary changes, data collection can begin. As mentioned previously, the fact-finding mission is the ultimate objective of the consultation process. How comfortable the patient is will make all the difference in the facts you uncover. Consultations can be done in many ways; none of them are right or wrong, and part of the consultations process will change based on the patient and his or her individual needs. Find the best one for the facility footprint and the clinicians in the practice. The process is really all about what makes sense for the facility, the physician, and the clinicians. Most of the time, consultation appointments are worked into the schedule around other appointments based on the needs for facility efficiencies and personnel availability. Rarely, if ever, do we think about how the patient might perceive the process and what might make the patient feel more comfortable.

Telephone Manners

Understanding why proper manners are a long lost art is difficult, but they are. Using the telephone properly, being polite, and making a patient feel important are concepts that are necessary to be successful and maintain a competitive edge. The fact is that the telephone is how nearly 100 percent of your patients make their first appointment, and it is how they often make follow-up appointments. In short, the telephone is how your customer will communicate with your company. If you think the front desk is not important, you should try to run a practice that has no telephone. A recent survey actually stated

> The consultation is an important meeting. During this time, the patient develops perceptions about your clinic, evaluates you as a clinician, and makes the active choice to return to the clinic.

that 49 percent of the complaints in the medical office related to telephone rudeness: long hold times, unreturned phone calls, and voicemail mazes.[2] Forty-nine percent is a big percentage of complaints directed at one specific area. Obviously, proper training and hiring will make a difference about how patients are treated. Training and hiring affects the capture rate of new patients and increases the return rate of established patients through telephones.

Potential new patients who are seeking information on the telephone can be classified into three categories: "knows what he or she wants," "needs information," and "is a price shopper." The person who knows what he or she wants has already done the investigation and is ready to make an appointment. Only the most rude and inept front desk person can dissuade this prospective client from making the appointment. The caller who needs information requires time and lots of it. This prospective client will be asking questions that cannot be answered over the telephone, and the objective of the front desk is to give as much information as possible without making it necessary for this future client to avoid an appointment. We will talk a little more about this patient in a moment. Finally, the price shopper may or may not make an appointment and is driven strictly by the price quote. All patients require proper telephone etiquette and manners because you never know who is going to book an appointment or if your pleasant demeanor is the driving reason why (Table 4–2).

Answering the Telephone

What is the proper way to answer the telephone? Our tendency, especially with multiple ringing lines, is to be quick and curt, and it begs the

Table 4–2   Good Telephone Manners

Right Thing to Say	Wrong Thing to Say
Thank you for calling. I can help answer your questions.	I am sorry, no one is here to answer your questions. Please call back.
I can give a price range.	We do not give prices over the telephone.
We provide many treatments that may meet your needs.	I do not know what treatments will work for you.
May I offer you a consultation with our clinician?	The clinician can call you back.

old joke, "If these patients would just leave us alone, we could get so much accomplished!" However, our telephone is our business. The proper greeting is: "Good morning, [name of company], this is [employee name]." Another welcome option is: "Thank you for calling [name of company], this is [employee name]. How may I help you today?" Either greeting is warm and inviting and encourages your caller to engage in conversation. All employees using the telephone should express themselves clearing and speak loudly (without yelling) and without mumbling. Do not speak to others in the office when you are also speaking on the telephone; this is rude. If you need to speak with a co-worker, put the patient on hold, and then return to the telephone when the conversation is finished. Remember, the person on the other end of the telephone cannot see your face. Your voice has to say it all. Make it good. Finally, answer the telephone on the first or second ring. If you must place someone on hold, ask his or her permission first. Transferring to the voicemail is one of the common options today. Make sure the caller is agreeable with this option and that this is not the third or fourth time that the caller has been placed into voicemail without a return call.

Returning Telephone Calls

All telephone calls should be returned as soon as possible, even though this is easier said than done. Although the reasons are many that telephone calls are left until the following day or not returned at all, bear in mind that this call is not only a prospective patient, but is also business. Failure to return telephone calls communicates a lack of caring and therefore unimportance. Do not give your caller this message.

Telephone Consultations

Many patients require a version of the telephone consultation; the caller who needs information will be the one who requires your time, patience, and energy. As a new patient, he or she will need to have many questions answered such as, "Is this treatment right for me?" "How many treatments will I need?" "How much improvement will I see?" All of these questions are difficult to answer over the telephone. This caller will also be skittish about scheduling an appointment. He or she will worry that the treatment is inappropriate. Patience! Help the caller get all of the answers to his or her questions in a sensitive and gentle manner; the caller just needs your help and support. If you get on the telephone with a person such as this, let your co-workers know you will be busy for a while and that you cannot be interrupted, which will help you concentrate on the caller and ensure the information you are giving is accurate and informative (Table 4–3).

Table 4–3 Objectives of a Telephone Consultation

Common Questions on the Telephone	Answers to the Questions	Objective of the Answer
What treatment is right for me?	Several treatments might work for you. The proper treatment will be determined at your consultation and after your skin is examined.	To help the patient understand that a skin consultation is necessary to answer the question accurately.
My friend had a treatment that she liked. I want that treatment too.	If your skin type is similar and the treatment is appropriate, the same treatment may be recommended.	Gently communicate that she is special and that the treatments will be just as effective, but for her.
How many treatments will I need to get rid of my hyperpigmentation?	That will be determined at your consultation, after a skin analysis.	Help the patient understand that a consultation is required.
How much will all of the necessary products cost?	The average cost for our therapeutic products runs about [your estimate] and lasts about [your estimate on usage]. Obviously, some products such as cleansers run out more quickly.	Just give general figures in this answer. You do not know what will be required.
Will the treatment hurt?	Everyone has a different pain tolerance; but the treatments are generally not uncomfortable.	Once again, give general answers. Everyone is special and different.
Who will do the treatment?	It depends on the type of procedure you are having. If you are having injection therapy such as Botox®, the nurse or physician will provide the treatment. If, on the other hand, you will be having a skin treatment, the aesthetician will provide that treatment.	Give the general guidelines for treatment in your facility.

Continued

Table 4–3   Objectives of a Telephone Consultation–Cont'd

How long will the consultation last?	We normally schedule [length of time]. If you have a lot of questions, perhaps we should schedule extra time.	Give her a good estimate of time. Remember, underpromise and overachieve.
Can my friend come with me?	Your consultation is a personal discussion about you, your health, and your skin care. Just be sure you do not mind disclosing personal information with your friend present.	Communicate the importance of privacy and our concern for her privacy.

Telephone consultations are the beginning of the patient-caregiver relationship and should not be considered a burden or hassle, just the opposite. The telephone consultation, whether short or long, will be the beginning of a patient relationship and should be handled with care.

> The objective of a telephone consultation is to set up an office consultation.

USING PSYCHOLOGIC AND COMMUNICATION CUES TO OPTIMIZE PERFORMANCE

Because people generally like to talk about themselves, and the consultation is no different, reviewing new patient documentation is a good time to build rapport with a patient. Use this opportunity as an icebreaker to get to know the patient. If your patient is shy or embarrassed, using this technique will help him or her get comfortable with you and the informational exchange.

Gauging a Patient's Commitment

Sometimes, the caller is on a fact-finding mission and is not yet ready to make a commitment to skin-care treatment or cosmetic surgery. These callers should be "handled" with the same amount of care as you would the patient who is obviously anxious and ready to begin care. The patient who is at the beginning stages of data collection will remember the good experiences and the poor experiences. If your office is the first one the person has visited, you will have a greater impact than the second or third office. The person is probably a little nervous, and your ability to put him or her at ease, answer his or her questions, and take him or her through a simple process will affect the impressions of you. The person is trying to make a decision, and you want him or her to make a decision to be your client.

Remember that first impressions are lasting impressions. Research tells us that only three seconds is needed to be appraised.[3] Just as you are evaluating your patient, he or she is evaluating you. Aside from appearance, the patient will be appraising you for your comfort zone in the business (i.e., *what you know, how knowledgeable you are*), whether a rapport will be established, and whether he or she will be able to communicate with you in a meaningful way.

Similarly, you will be gauging the prospective patient. Does he or she appear to be of a class that can afford your services? Is he or she well groomed? Are you intrigued by him or her, or have you written this person off, after three seconds?[4] These thoughts can be interesting. Do you write off your prospective patients, close their wallets, and generally disregard them before they even get to your treatment room? If you do, then you may find that your patient list is short and diminishing by the day.

Do not be misled by patient appearances; listen to what the patient is saying to you. The patient sometimes does not know what he or she wants, and figuring out how the caller will be helped the most will be up to you (Table 4–4).

Problem-Oriented Consultations

When problems arise, or when a plateau is reached in the care, a consultation to discuss the patient's status is a good idea. Be

Table 4–4 Gauging Patient Commitment

Behaviors that Demonstrate Commitment	Behaviors that Demonstrate a Lack of Commitment
Questions specific to the resolution of their condition	Concerned about the treatments and products
Comfortable with prices	Time constrained
Comfortable with treatment process	Budget constrained
Engaging and comfortable in the discussion	Discussion concerning lack of commitment Avoids eye contact

proactive if you sense unhappiness on the part of the patient. The objective of this consultation is to collect information that is specific to the care of the patient and how it is affecting the outcome. For example, a common problem-oriented consultation might involve the patient's perception of the result. Problem-oriented results have a different approach than that of traditional first-time consultations, but the mission is still a fact-finding mission. You will be asking in-depth questions about the home-care program and looking for problems that are affecting the result or process of home-care treatments.

A desire to blame someone is often found in a consultation that is associated with a patient problem. Either the patient will want to blame you, or you want to blame the patient. Try very hard to avoid these feelings. In fact, try to avoid your feelings all together. Your feelings have no place in this situation. Placing blame does not change the situation and can only lead to an unhappy discourse (Table 4–5).

Patient Frustrations with Consultations

Patients who have been interviewed about the frustrations of their consultations respond by listing some of the following: waiting too long, not having all their questions answered, rudeness (both at the front desk and by the clinical staff), feeling rushed, feeling "sold," and no rapport with the clinician (Table 4–6).

Body Dysmorphic Disorder

One of the more significant uses for communication and psychologic cues will be evaluating each patient for psychologic disorders such as

Table 4–5 Problem-Oriented Consultations

Patient Problem	Consultation Objective
Treatment is not progressing.	Understand why the treatment has met an impasse.
Treatment has complications.	Alleviate the complication, and sustain the patient relationship.
Patient is not following instructions.	Teach about the value of participation.

Table 4–6   Patient Frustrations With Consultations

Common Frustration	Source of the Frustration
Waiting	The clinic is overscheduled.
Questions not answered	The literature is not clear; not enough time during the consultation to answer questions.
Rudeness	Staff is inadequate or poorly trained.
Feeling rushed	The schedule is overbooked.
Feeling "sold"	The staff is too pushy during the education process.
No rapport	Communication clarity is lacking.

body dysmorphic disorder

A psychosocial disorder that causes individuals to be inappropriately concerned with their appearance. Persons affected with BDD are contraindicated for most aesthetic procedures.

body dysmorphic disorder (BDD). BDD is an emotional disorder that causes individuals to be inappropriately concerned with their appearance. People with BDD are focused on the appearance of their skin, hair, nose, or ears, in particular. They may have minor defects of the nose or small scars that they believe to be overwhelmingly obvious. Individuals with BDD are also concerned about their eyes, believing that their eyes are too small or otherwise unattractive. Persons with BDD spend at least 1 hour a day thinking negative thoughts about their appearance.

Not surprisingly, patients with BDD have difficulty in their social life or work life, or both. They often have difficulty meeting new people or making and keeping friends because they are so self-conscious about their appearance. They often spend time alone in their home, often alienating family or those who care about them. These patients may seem overly critical of their skin and appearance. Assuming that the patient is being treated by a psychiatrist, one of the easiest methods is to look at the medications that the client is taking. For persons under treatment, you will find a medication that is treating mood disorders. However, do not be mislead that not all clients who are on medication for mood disorders have BDD. If BDD is suspected, the clinician should simply ask the patient if he or she is afflicted with the disorder.

Red flags for BDD include depression, anxiety, acute stress, and obsessive and compulsive behavior.[5] Individuals with BDD will sometimes appear efficient and organized, but when the client is under stress, the previously subtle symptoms of BDD will become apparent.

Clients with BDD have a high incidence of dissatisfaction with results, and any small complication can cause undue stress for the clinician and client alike.[6] The most important question the clinician should be asking in situations in which BDD is suspected is, "Can I satisfy this client?" If the clinician has a concern about his or her ability to satisfy the patient, the client should be turned away or referred to the physician for further consultation.

> BDD can be subtle and difficult to detect. If you are unsure if your patient falls into this category, the patient should be referred to your clinic physician.

TOP TEN TIPS TO TAKE TO THE CLINIC

1. Be prepared for every consultation.
2. Each patient is different; therefore you will need to adjust your consultation to meet the patient's needs.
3. Use the knowledge of your team members to meet the needs of the patient.
4. Understand your role in the different consultative processes.
5. A consultation is a fact-finding mission for the clinician, but the patient must be made comfortable and able to trust.
6. Use the information sheets the patient fills out to your advantage.
7. Know the frustrations that patients can have with the consultation process.
8. Have professional telephone manners.
9. Know the objective of the telephone interview.
10. Be kind and thoughtful toward the patient.

CHAPTER REVIEW QUESTIONS

1. What is the objective of the consultative process?
2. How do you know if the patient is interested in the services discussed?
3. What is the objective of the telephone interview process?
4. Why is the patient scared during the consultation?
5. What are the symptoms of BDD?
6. What are the different types of consultations?
7. Why are team approaches to consultations important?

BIBLIOGRAPHY

ETICON, Inc. (2005, May 24). *Etiquette for business: What's rudeness costing you?* [Online]. Available: http://www.eticon.com

Lavington, C. (1997). *You've only got three seconds.* New York: Broadway Books Doubleday.

Leonardo, J. (2003, August). Negotiating the gray area of BDD and the bottom line. *Plastic Surgery News,* 14(8), 24.

The Body Dysmorphic Disorder Clinic and Research Unit. (2004, January 14). [On line]. Available: http://ww.massgeneral.org

CHAPTER REFERENCES

1. Lavington, C. (1997). *You've only got three seconds,* New York: Broadway Books Doubleday, New York, New York.

2. ETICON, Inc. (2005, May 24). *Etiquette for business: What's rudeness costing you?* [Online]. Available: http://www.eticon.com/rudeness.htm

3. Lavington, C. (1997). *You've only got three seconds,* Broadway Books Doubleday, New York, New York.

4. Lavington, C. (1997). *You've only got three seconds,* Broadway Books Doubleday, New York, New York.

5. Leonardo, J. (2003, August). Negotiating the gray area of BDD, and the bottom line. *Plastic Surgery News, Vol.* 14(8).

6. Massachusetts General Hospital. (2004, January 14). *The body dysmorphic clinic and research unit.* [On line]. Available: http://www.massgeneral.org

Treatment Plans

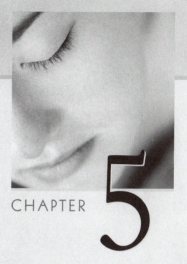

CHAPTER 5

LEARNING OBJECTIVES

After completing this chapter you should be able to:

1. Discuss the benefit of treatment care plans.
2. Describe the process of creating a treatment care plan.
3. Discuss patient education, behavior modification, social constraints, and budget matters, as well as how they affect the outcome of a treatment plan.

INTRODUCTION

O nce the data is collected from a consultation, what do you do with it? Write it down and forget about it? Many clinicians do. As we discussed in Chapter 4, the information you cull from the consultation is your opportunity for success or failure. The objective and subjective information that is gathered during a consultation should be turned into a document that can be used in a meaningful and proactive manner. In other words, put the information into a plan of action. For our purposes, we will refer to this plan of action as a **treatment plan**.

Creating a simple treatment plan is only a three-step process: data collection, problem identification, and a formulation of the plan. All three of these steps are interrelated and one cannot be done without the others. Additionally, the steps must occur in sequential order to be effective. Remember that this plan is collaborative and involves other members of the team. Therefore the steps for setting up the plan will be *multifactorial, multilayered*, and *multistaged*.

Writing a plan should be fast and easy. If it is made too complex, the process will not be used, and this important effort will fall by the wayside. The framework should be standardized with a form that all clinicians in the facility use. Remember, you will be assessing the patient, identifying the problem, making a plan, setting goals, implementing the plan, and evaluating the results. More than likely, you take all of these steps right now. What you gain by writing the process down is creating a paper trail, the ability to communicate with the patient more effectively, efficient planning and goal setting, and a more sophisticated method of evaluation. It creates clarity for the patient and a superior treatment model for the clinic.

treatment plan
A plan of action for patient care.

DEFINING THE TREATMENT PLAN

A concise definition of the treatment plan is a document that will create the pathway for positive outcomes and increased patient satisfaction. The treatment plan benefits the patient, the individual clinician, and the clinic. For the components of the plan to fall into place, all parties must be involved. For the process to function smoothly, examining the process from a top-down perspective makes good sense.

To work from a top-down prospective, you will need to ask broad questions that will give you more specific details about the patient, the treatments preferred, and the goals of treatment. The first step in setting up a care plan is data collection. We have spent a good deal of time talking about the consultation and different ways to collect data. Not enough can be said about good data collection. As you now see, data collection is the backbone of the process, and without a solid consultation, a useful treatment plan will not unfold. However, as previously discussed, collecting data is a fine art and one that should not appear as *data collection*. Remember that the comfort and emotional safety of the patient is important if you are going to be successful in this process. To best accomplish this task, you will want to ask yourself the right questions during data collection: who, what, when, where, and how. Let us delve into these questions. The ability to answer the questions in a meaningful way will contribute to your success in treatment plan development.

Who

First is the question of *who*. When you ask yourself *who*, you should address the following questions: "Who gets a treatment plan?" "Who will be conducting the treatments outlined in the treatment plan?"

First, do you need a formalized treatment plan? The answer is "yes," in some fashion either lengthy or abbreviated, every patient needs a treatment plan. Patients who come to the clinic with long-term multilayer problems must have a treatment plan that focuses on the end point or goal of the treatment. These treatment plans will be detailed and explain the short- and long-term agenda the clinician has for the patient and the objective of care. Patients with simpler problems may require only brief treatment plans.

Next, *who* will be treated? At this point, you evaluate the individual patient, his or her goals, and his or her expectations. When a patient first comes to a spa or clinic, he or she has a set of goals and expectations that may or may not coincide with your capabilities or the capabilities of the procedures you have to offer. The manner in which you manage your patient's knowledge level and expectations will be a critical component to your ability to be successful. Reeducating the patients to prevent disappointment will be to your advantage.

Finally, *who* will be conducting the treatments? Because of variant degrees of certification and expertise, different staff members may be needed to perform certain procedures with a particular patient. One of the important processes that should be in place at the facility is that of interoffice referral patterns and the success that clinicians have referring back and forth to each other. This process should be dictated by a treatment plan and put in motion by the primary clinician.

What

What are we treating? This category should answer all of the diagnostic questions, such as **dyschromias**, solar damage, or acne, in other words, identifying *what* the problem is. In many cases, the problems will be multilayered and multifactorial. For example, the patient presents with hyperpigmentation but is also on birth control pills, which may be contributing to the dyschromias. The patient does not want to go off the birth control pill but would like to improve her skin. This caveat needs to be included in the treatment plan. More commonly, the patient may be seeking antiaging solutions. These patients often have dyschromias and skin laxity, as well as **dynamic rhytids** and **static rhytids**. These multifactorial problems require multifactorial solutions and team coordination. Obviously, this factor is at the core of the treatment plan.

When

When should answer the questions of when the treatments will begin. Remembering that these problems can be multilayered, the focus of the treatments will be determined on the priorities that the clinician and the patient have discussed. When should also encompass the time frame required to complete the stated goals, which will be detailed in the treatment plan.

Where

Where should answer all of the questions about the treatment logistics. Where might mean not only the *where* in the facility, but also the *where* on the body. Being specific when you state the locations of problem areas or treatment targets is to your advantage. Instead of saying "treating lines on the face," you should refer to specific areas on the face so as to minimize miscommunications. For example, "treat fine lines of the glabella and crow's feet." Policy and procedures should be in place to guide the clinician through this component of the treatment plan.

How

How is the bulk of the plan but does not come into focus without the aforementioned questions answered. *How* should relate to the process of program implementation. If the program is going to include multiple clinicians, a written calendar should outline the proposed plan and when certain procedures are to take place. For example, does Botox® treatment occur before starting a microdermabrasion program, or how soon after the start of the home-care program can the clinical treatments begin?

Treatment Plans and Medical Legal Issues

The treatment plan may not be the most important form of protection for the clinician when it comes to medical legal issues, but it still plays a valuable role. The rule of thumb in medical charting is: *if it is not written in the chart, it did not happen.* A properly documented treatment plan will organize and outline the care for the patient. This approach will be helpful if you should ever need to defend your position regarding the discussions you had with the patient and any recommended course of action. The document should outline the patient's responsibilities: application of home-care products and making and keeping appointments. The treatment plan also directs the staff's actions and creates a pathway of care that should be followed. Any changes in care should be clearly and concisely documented. The documentation should include reasons for the changes, who dictated the changes, the patient's response to and participation in the changes, and, of course, the new treatment plan.

■ DEVELOPING A TREATMENT PLAN

The next step is to understand the problem and to be able to articulate in the treatment plan the specific problems. This step is sometimes easier said than done. The clinician must listen carefully during the consultation, take notes, and create priorities. The clinician must also know how to ask relevant questions. These priorities and the interpretation of the data must be discussed with the patient to ensure that your interpretation is the same as his or hers. Additionally, several problems may be emanating from a variety of factors, which will make the process harder. Nevertheless, all of the problems should be identified and documented, whether currently pertinent to the patient or not (refer to sample form on page 76). A common example might be that a patient is concerned about dyschromias, but under the discoloration is **telangiectasia**. Although the telangiectasia is not important to the patient while the discoloration is present, it will be after the dyschromias has cleared. Pointing out such problems and documenting accordingly is up to the clinician.

telangiectasia
Small visible capillaries sometimes referred to as broken capillaries.

Once you have garnered the necessary answers to these questions, the treatment plan can now be established. Although all of the information is important, the most critical will be the answers to the following questions: "What are the goals of treatment?" "What treatments will be used to achieve the goal?" "What is the timetable involved in accomplishing as much?" These areas of the treatment plan bring back into focus for both the clinician and the patient, specifically, "what we are

Treatment Plan

Date: _____

Patient Name: _____

Patient complaints:

- Aging
- Pigmentation
- Telangiectasia
- Acne
- Scars
- Postsurgical complications

Contributing factors to current condition:

- No sunscreen
- Medications
- Poor home-care program
- Genetics

Clinician conclusions:

_____

_____

Treatment plan:

- Glycolic acid peels
- Jessner's peels
- Trichloracetic acid or Obagi® peels
- Foto Facial®
- Microdermabrasion
- Dermal fillers
- Botox®
- Laser hair removal
- Facials
- Waxing and tinting

Number of treatments:

- 3–5 every other week, then monthly
- 6–10 every other week, then monthly
- Monthly
- Bi-monthly

Treatment Plan—cont'd

Rationale:

_____
_____
_____

Goal:

_____
_____
_____

Participating clinicians:

- Aesthetician
- Registered nurse injector
- Physician

Desired outcome:

_____
_____

---

going to do." Each problem should have a treatment. All problems are interrelated to the final goal: skin care, antiaging, and injectables. Therefore all of the treatments should be discussed.

Although we want the patient to participate in the care plan, allowing the patient to have a direct hand in the development of the treatment plan may not be exceptionally wise, by this statement we mean the ability to control the types of procedures that are recommended or the products that are recommended. Do not be misled; the patient has every right to decide whether he or she will or will not participate in the outlined program. However, developing the plan and getting the patient to accept the program would be wise for the clinician. Allowing the patient to direct the plan creates all kinds of potential problems, including accountability and efficacy.

Evaluating Patient Concerns

The first section involves patient concerns. This information is what the patient has told you about the reason for his or her visit, that is, the exact nature of the problem as the patient sees it. This information should be written on the treatment plan exactly as it is communicated to you. Patients can be very descriptive about their problems. Getting some exact quotes in this section will be helpful to both you and the patient as you revisit this document in later months.

Evaluating Contributing Factors

Contributing factors are issues that have made the condition what it is today and how behavior modification will play into the treatment plan. For example, if the patient is a smoker, this may be problematic if upper lip lines and facial aging are the focus, in addition to, of course, the patient's general health. Another example might be patients who refuse to wear sunscreen on the face. These examples cause **extrinsic aging** and can be limited with a change in habits. Other problems may be thin, transparent skin or lines above the lip that are unrelated to smoking. These factors are defined as **intrinsic aging**. When documenting the contributing factors, a causal relationship should be noted (Tables 5-1 and 5-2).

Drawing Conclusions

Clinician conclusions is the section in which you give your opinion. This area is where your analysis and assessment of the skin, the patient, and the current situation belong. The clinician should focus on statements that contain language such as "patient states" or "skin appears to be." Although the clinician may know exactly what the problems are and how they came to be, making a true clinical diagnosis is inappropriate for the

extrinsic aging
Changes that are brought on by the effects of the environment and our choices relating to them, specifically sunlight exposure.

intrinsic aging
Changes that would occur over time without the effects of any environmental factors.

Table 5–1   Important Information Necessary to Create the Treatment Plan

Important Information	Form	Other Data Sources	Use
Current medications	Health form	Discussion with patient	Evaluating for photosensitive drugs or other medications that will interfere with treatment
Current health problems	Health form	Discussion with patient	Evaluating for illness that may contraindicate the patient for treatment
Current skin problems	Skin health form	Discussion with patient	Looking for the current skin problems: acne, dyschromias, solar damage, and so forth
Skin goals	Skin health form	Discussion with patient	Evaluating mutual goals with the patient
Long-term aesthetic goals	Skin health form	Discussion with patient	Evaluating mutual goals with the patient
Skin-care habits	Skin health form	Discussion with patient	Understanding what the patient does now and what can be expected in terms of behavior changes
Budget restraints		Discussion with patient	Building an effective plan with budget issues in mind, if necessary

Table 5–2 Three Steps to Building a Treatment Plan

	Data Collection	Problem Identification	Plan of Action
Information on forms filled out by the patient	X	X	
Patient's short-term goals	X	X	
Patient's long-term goals	X		X

clinician. This diagnostic determination is for the physician only. There-fore carefully word your language, including the critical information.

Determining the Number of Treatments

Under the heading *number of treatments,* the clinician should identify for each recommended treatment the estimated number of treatments that will be necessary to achieve the goal. This process may be complex if the program recommends several different treatments. In this case, making specific notes relating to each procedure will be necessary.

Participating Staff Members

Typically more than one clinician will be working with the patient. At least two will be involved in implementing the plan, depending on the chosen plan of action. If possible, the patient should see the same clinicians for the same treatment. This process creates consistency.

This section should reflect all the clinicians that are expected to participate in the patient's care. If the patient will be seeing a nurse or physician for dermal fillers or Botox®, the appointment or consultation should be noted in the treatment plan. Additionally, if different clinicians provide different treatments, such as facials, hair removal laser, or microdermabrasion, all the clinicians should be noted. If possible, specific recommendations should be made, which will help the patient know for whom to ask when making appointments. Research shows that the more team members that participate in the patient care, the higher the satisfaction rate will be among patients. So make the care a team effort.

Patient Education and Behavior Modification

Patient education is one of the most important elements for success in a program. The patient-education program involves two areas. First is the home-care program: how to use it, why it is important, and how the patient is responsible for the ultimate result based on the program. The second component of the educational process is for the patient to understand the scope of the program. In this arm of the education, the clinician must help the patient understand the entire program: home-care and clinical factors and how each of these elements affects the skin. Hence a brief understanding of the skin itself is necessary. In some cases, the patient will not be interested in this information. The clinician will need to customize the educational program for the patient, focusing on the result and the end point.

The treatment plan is often used as a framework for communication. This document, when it is done well, will help the clinician communicate the plan, reintroduce the patient to his or her goals, and keep the program moving forward. Getting a patient to move forward and to make commitments in *small steps* rather than *large leaps* is always easier; the treatment plan will help you accomplish this task for your patient. As a communication tool, the document will help keep the patient focused on the outcome and the process. In many ways, the document takes away from some of the "nagging" in which clinicians find themselves involved: getting patients to comply with the home-care program and completing the treatment plan.

The treatment plan helps identify the behaviors you will need to help the patient modify, for example, wearing sunscreen. Remember that behavior modification requires education. Developing the necessary relationship and beginning the educational process with the patient will take time, but it will be the backbone of the success of the program. Therefore, in the beginning, you may want to plan extra time at each appointment to bond with the patient and provide some education.

IMPLEMENTING THE TREATMENT PLAN

The last stage of the process is the actual implementation. Given that most of the plans you create will be used by multiple caretakers, care should be taken to describe all of the actions necessary to treat the identified problems. The treatment plan itself needs to be "specific, realistic, measurable, have a definite time frame to achieve the result, considerate of the patient's desires."[1] Implementing the plan is really simply taking care of the patient in an orderly fashion, with treatment rationale, goals, and evaluation of the result.

Communication of Treatment Rationale

Rationale is a new concept for most clinicians and will be difficult for the clinician initially. Just remember, the rationale refers to the *why* of the treatment plan, in others word, *why* a microdermabrasion and not a peel. The *why* helps you assess the correctness of the treatment and will be part of the evaluation of the success of the program. If you happen to vary from the treatment plan—and this will happen based on the condition of the patient's skin—you need a rationale documented in the chart.

Communication of Goals

Goals define the steps of the program: where are we going, and how will we know when we get there? Mini-goals should be set in the program that will show that gains are being made. The goals (and results) should be discussed with the patient on a regular basis, and new goals should be set, when appropriate.

Managing Patient Care

The process we have been discussing is one that is managed by the skin-care clinician. This person creates the plan, monitors it, and evaluates the success. However, this model is not true for every facility. In some clinics, the physician or nurse is responsible for the creation, guidance, and direction of the treatment plan. Regardless of who creates or manages the plan, many members of the team are involved. An important point to remember is your individual responsibility to the patient and the team. Communicating and documenting the patient's progress and making recommendations to update the treatment plan will ensure that the goals that have been set will be achieved.

Social and Business Constraints

Many times, the patient will have constraints around which the clinician will need to work to achieve the desired result. Most patients are sensitive about how they look. Obviously, this reason is why they came to the clinic! Their schedules may dictate how and when the treatments are performed. Many times, patients do not want others to know about their treatments, and therefore the idea of being red or "peely" will be a deterrent for care and treatment. The clinician must work around the patient's schedule and be sure that their appearance needs can be met. Ensuring that this goal is satisfactorily met will require education, proper home-care products, and good makeup. Each of these factors will play a role to ensure the best appearance for the patient.

Patient's Budget

One of the most important aspects of ensuring success for the patient is working within his or her budget. Some patients will not have budgetary issues, but many will. Setting up a budget in advance may be comforting to patients, even those who can easily afford your services. This issue is best discussed in advance, whether by the clinician or the business manager, to ensure that no misunderstandings develop once the patient has embarked on the treatment program. If breaking down the treatment plan and products into a monthly amount is possible, the process will be more easily understood and accepted. Additionally, if you have a form on which to write it down, it will help create clarity. Even though most spas or medical spas have a menu of services, which is a great place to start, taking it one step further will help the patient understand the financial commitment. Once the patient has gotten past the financial hurdle, keeping the patient focused on the goals and results of his or her skin care is much easier.

▪ EVALUATION OF THE TREATMENT PLAN

Evaluating the success of a plan may be difficult, given the number of ways to interpret success. This aspect is one of the benefits of the treatment plan. The plan should be outlined before treatment begins and updated as the care continues. That said, the clinician might want to use advanced tools to determine the success of the treatment plan. Among these tools are retention rates, referral rates, referral categories, and patient feedback.

Evaluating the retention rate is the most logical determination of success aside from the actual plan analysis. In other words, is the patient returning for treatment? This information may be extrapolated to happy, satisfied patients. Referral rates are also an indication of happy, satisfied patients. Patients who refer friends are often happy and satisfied with treatment and results. Referral categories are also an indicator of specific patient happiness. In other words, the patient's friends are referred for skin care but not for Botox®. Finally, patient feedback is also valuable. Obtaining information from patients can be done in many ways. First, patients who complain should be rewarded. These patients make your practice continue to improve because they took the time to complain. Other ways to mine for patient feedback include questionnaire cards or surveys and outbound manager calls (Table 5–3).

Table 5–3 Tools Used to Evaluate Success

Tool	How to Use It	What It Will Show
Retention rates	Evaluate the clinician's ability to retain patients.	Happy and satisfied patients
Referral rates	Track referrals each month.	Shows increases in referral rates and reflects happy and satisfied patients
Referral categories	Referrals are broken down into categories. The most important category is patients who refer other patients.	Communicates happy and satisfied patients who are willing to refer
Patient feedback	Use survey cards, telephone calls, and questionnaires.	Reflects happy and satisfied patients as well as other valuable feedback

Goals

Staying motivated and excited by a treatment plan is easier for both the patient and the clinician if goals are in place. Initially, goals such as mastering the home-care program, for example, will be easy to reach. As time goes on, the goals will become more challenging. Nevertheless, the goals should be achievable. Remember that goals need to be flexible, fluid, and constantly reviewed. Goals might change if the patient's needs or objectives have evolved. Goals might also change to reflect advanced improvement in the patient's progress or the addition of new therapies and added technology.

Desired Outcomes

The desired outcome is the end result: what we hope to achieve for the patient. The desired outcome is far reaching and discusses goals and objectives. This document represents, in fact, the long-range plan that may take years to achieve. As is the case in many examples we have mentioned, the desired outcome may be multifactorial and multilayered. A long-term desired outcome may involve a patient behavior modification goal (the use of sunscreen), the treatment of dyschromias and telangiectasia, followed by **glabella** line treatment, and, over time, followed by facelift surgery. This example is, of course, multifactorial, multilayered and multiclinician focused; but then, most outcomes are.

glabella

The area of skin between the eyebrows, the underlying muscle groups of which cause creasing, or "frown lines," as a result of repeated squinting or frowning over time.

Critical Thinking

Critical thinking is an important component of developing a treatment plan. Critical thinking is defined as the "intellectually disciplined process of actively and skillfully conceptualizing, applying, analyzing, synthesizing, and evaluating information gathered from or generated by observation, experience, reflection, reasoning, or communication as a guide to belief and action."[2]

The ability to be a critical thinker is a valuable tool when working in the medical spa, whether we are discussing treatment plans or other areas of performance. The capacity to collect information and use it in a meaningful way to improve the status of the patient is among the most valuable skills.

Conclusion

Using a treatment plan for the care of the nonsurgical aesthetic patient requires knowledge of the patient, the process, and the participation of all members of the team. The document must be focused on the activities that will need to occur for the patient to achieve the desired goals. Furthermore, clinicians should be trained in the use of the document, and random chart checks should be done to ensure that the process is properly advancing. Additionally, management must make the process accessible for the clinician. In other words, how does the schedule work? Will it allow for the proper use of the document? If not, how will processes be changed to accommodate this update in patient care?

Although none of these steps will be easy, the effort will be worthwhile. Clinicians who use these documents and processes find an organized, thoughtful patient care course. Communication between clinicians and medical professionals is increased, and patient satisfaction is enhanced.

▶ ›› TOP TEN TIPS TO TAKE TO THE CLINIC

1. Make a comfortable consultation and treatment room, which will help the patient share information.
2. Treatment plans are multifactorial, multilayered, and multiclinician.
3. Create forms for the patient to complete that capture the information you are looking to use in a treatment plan.

4. Always use critical thinking.
5. Three simple steps are involved in completing a treatment plan. Use them in sequential order.
6. Be sure that each step of the plan is complete and that the other members of the team are aware of their role in the patient's care.
7. Education of the patient is key to the success of the program.
8. Behavior modification will always be necessary.
9. Respect the patient's budget.
10. Treatment plans are part of the legal document known as the *chart*.

CHAPTER REVIEW QUESTIONS

1. What information should be found at the consultation?
2. What is the purpose of a treatment plan?
3. What are the steps to develop a treatment plan?
4. Who are the professionals who participate in a treatment plan and therefore the care of the patient?
5. How does the patient's current skin-care habits affect the treatment plan?
6. Why is critical thinking important to the development of the treatment plan?
7. Why is patient retention important when evaluating a treatment plan?

BIBLIOGRAPHY

The Body Dysmorphic Disorder Clinic and Research Unit. (2004, January 14). [Online]. Available: *http://www.massgeneral.org*

Deitz, S. (2004). *Milady's the clinical esthetician.* Clifton Park, NY: Thomson Delmar Learning.

Doenges, M., Moorhouse, M. F., & Murr-Geissler, A. (2002). *Nursing care plans: Guidelines for individualizing patient care.* Philadelphia: F. A. Davis.

Leonardo, J. (2003, August). Negotiating the gray area of BDD, and the bottom line. *Plastic Surgery News,* 14(8), 24.

Merriam-Webster's Collegiate Dictionary. (1992). New York: Random House.

Wilhelm, S. (2004, January 14). *Body dysmorphic disorder clinic and research unit* [Online]. Available: http://www.mgh.harvard.edu

CHAPTER REFERENCES

1. Doenges, M., Moorhouse, M. F., & Murr-Geissler, A. (2002). *Nursing care plans: Guidelines for individualizing patient care.* Philadelphia: F. A. Davis.
2. Doenges, M. Moorhouse, M. F., & Murr-Geissler, A. (2002). *Nursing care plans: Guidelines for individualizing patient care.* Philadelphia: F. A. Davis.

Complications, Side Effects, and Consequences of Treatment

CHAPTER 6

KEY TERMS

complications	side effects
self-aware	treatment consequences

LEARNING OBJECTIVES

After completing this chapter you should be able to:

1. Define complications, side effects, and consequences.
2. Understand the difference among complications, side effects, and consequences.
3. Understand the physical healing of complications, side effects, and consequences.
4. Explain the emotional healing of complications, side effects, and consequences.

INTRODUCTION

Now that the treatment plan has been completed, the outlined procedures can now be enacted. All clinicians fear that they will make a mistake and cause complications for their patients; and yet, the odds are that this event will not happen. Moreover, the events that we see in the medical spa are not truly complications but rather are consequences of treatment or side effects of treatment. What then constitutes a complication, and how is this different from a side effect or a treatment consequence? We hear these words used all of the time, but are they used in the correct context and for the right reason? In fact, significant differences exist between a complication and a treatment consequence. For clinicians working in the medical spa, knowing and understanding the differences among these three labels is important.

Complications are unexpected events that occur following a normally applied procedure. For example, a patient has a peel, and a scar results.

Side effects are "an action or effect of a drug other than that desired, such as nausea or vomiting."[1] In the case of medical skin care, an example might be dry and irritated skin while using Retin A® or glycolic acid.

Treatment consequences are predictable outcomes of the procedure that occur in a reasonable percentage of people having the procedure. In other words, a patient has a light peel, and superficial "rug burns" result.

That said, let us move on and discuss in detail situations in each category and what to do, if anything, about them.

complications
Unexpected events that occur following a normally applied procedure.

side effects
An action or effect of a drug other than that desired, such as nausea or vomiting.

treatment consequences
Predictable outcomes of the procedure that occur in a reasonable percentage of people having the procedure.

▪ COMPLICATIONS

The word complications can tie the clinician's stomach in knots. Nothing rings fear as much as a complication. In fact, the word complication often describes a mishap or *problem.*

However, let us bring some reality to the situation. What really constitutes a complication in the world of medical microdermabrasion, peeling, and medical skin care? These procedures are safe and rarely have complications. In the medical spa, the only *real* complications are infection, scarring, and eye damage from either crystals or peel solutions in the eyes. All other events are qualified as treatment consequences or side effects.

Complications, if they occur, can be minimized for the clinician and patient by following a number of steps. Among the important first steps is the clinician's response. Does he or she panic and refuse to speak to the patient, or does the clinician respond appropriately? Next is patient education. Fear of the unknown can exacerbate the complication. Make sure the patient understands the problem and the options for solutions. Communication in these situations is critical. The clinician should bring the physician and the practice manager into the situation, if necessary. However, keep the lines of communication open. The clinician should be well schooled in understanding that the patient will have predictable responses. Be prepared for the patient and his or her responses. The patient will go through not only a physical healing, but also an emotional healing. Allow the patient the space and opportunity to go through this process with dignity.

Clinician Response to Complications of Treatment

Any clinician, nurse, or physician can tell you, when a complication occurs, you can see your career flash before your eyes. What if the patient becomes irreparably damaged? What if you get fired? What will happen to your insurance rates? What if you get sued? Although the possibility of these things happening is real, taking proactive steps during the consultation, and realizing quickly that a complication has occurred, will minimize this likelihood. Communication is the key to successful damage control. First, make sure, before treatment begins, that the patient is informed of the risks. The patient and the clinician should sign a treatment consent, which outlines the possible complications. This step is important in the communication process with the patient. Second, you should know the processes that should be in place in the event of a complication. For example, you should know from whom to seek help in your place of employment. Attempting to correct a situation for which you are not trained or ignoring early symptoms of a complication might be considered gross negligence. If a complication occurs, be compassionate and sympathetic to the patient's feelings; doing so will be of utmost importance. Effective management of complications will depend heavily on the steps you take both before and at the earliest stages of the complication.

Patient Education

We have already discussed the value of patient education. In the context of a complication, education is that much more important. During the consultative course of your interaction with a patient, you should have discussed the treatment you have recommended to realize the patient's particular goals. An important addendum to this discussion should include the risk associated with the treatment.

Your initial feelings might be to withhold this information for fear of scaring the patient away. Certainly, hearing that scarring or tissue damage may result will be frightening to many people, and it may, in fact, scare some people away. However, communicating this possibility has a dual benefit. First, when a complication does not occur, which ideally should be the vast majority of the time, the patient will have greater faith in your professional capacities for avoiding any aforementioned complications. Second, if a complication does occur, managing for the patient is psychologically easier if he or she is prepared for this possibility.

Of course, patient education is one of the most important aspects of patient care. The more accurate information the patient has, the better prepared they will be for the healing course. This process can be accomplished in a variety of ways, and multiple techniques should be used to ensure that the patient understands the information. In general, the common sources include printed literature, videos, the Internet, face-to-face discussion through an organized consultation process, consent forms, and patient referrals. Each of these sources has value and should be considered when educating patients.

Printed literature is probably the most common approach used to improve patient knowledge. The approach allows patients to take information, read it, and make a list of relevant questions for the clinician. Literature that is specific to the procedure and your facility orients the patient to the clinic's thinking and processes. This knowledge eliminates misunderstandings such as, "My girlfriend said the procedure would be done this way" or "In the other clinic I went to they did it this way." Additionally, literature burdens the patient with some responsibility to read and evaluate the information before taking part in the procedure or procedures.

Videos are a common product used to educate patients, especially in the cosmetic plastic surgery office. Videos are available from manufacturers that show procedures and discuss procedure consequences and complications. The combination of a video and literature can be the best training tools available, especially for medical microdermabrasion. However, the need for the clinician to *talk* to the client is not eliminated!

The Internet can be a good place for patients to do primary research on procedures they are considering. Aside from your own web site, refer the patient to additional web addresses that provide accurate educational material. A *third-party opinion* can be valuable in the educational process.

All of the previously mentioned sources should be used in concert with a face-to-face consultation. Not enough can be said about the value of an organized and informational consultation. As you already now know, the consultation is not only about educating the patient, but also about creating a bond.

Communication and Complications

Fair, honest, and compassionate communication is one of the most important skills you will use during a complication and the subsequent associated healing process. Becoming defensive during an event such as a complication is so easy for the clinician, and this is the last behavior that we want to exhibit. Therefore exactly what is fair, honest, and compassionate communication?

Management guru Peter Drucker makes the best statement about communication, and it is applicable to this situation: "I no longer think that learning how to manage other people, especially subordinates, is the most important thing for executives to learn. I am teaching, above all, how to manage oneself."[2] The secret to fair, honest, and compassionate communication is the ability to manage one's self. The best communication comes with the ability to be **self-aware** and able to assess the situation fairly without the emotional attachment. These concepts are fairly esoteric, and in these situations, we need tools to keep emotions in check. Therefore consider the following concepts. Poor communication may result when the sender has a poor working knowledge of the subject. In other words, you do not understand the complication and are frightened by the situation. Initially, this situation may be the one in which you find yourself. Do not communicate your fear to the patient. Find your clinic physician or the appropriate co-worker to help you speak with the patient. If you are afraid, the patient will be afraid. Do not let the patient sense your fear. Poor communication may also be the result of your lack of belief in the message. For example, you tell the patient that scarring will not occur, yet you believe it might or will scar. Poor communication also happens when the receiver is not paying attention, for example if the patient is looking in the mirror rather than listening to you. Finally, the concept of respect plays into the situation. If the patient does not respect you and will not listen to you, turning the care over to a co-worker will be in the patient's best interest. You can continue to follow the patient, but bow out gracefully.

self-aware
The ability to assess the situation without the emotional attachment.

Patient Responses to Complications of Treatment

As you know, complications of treatment are events that are not the expected results of a treatment. For example, a patient comes in for a dermal filler treatment; a tissue necrosis occurs followed by a scar. Patients will often have a wide variety of reactions to complications, from anger to fright. Initially, the patient will seemly accept the potential complication with ease and understanding. However, as the healing continues and the office visits become numerous, the patient may become angry. This reaction is common. A female patient will often use her boyfriend or husband as a weapon. ''My husband is really angry at this situation.'' Complications can often be exacerbated by personal relationships. A husband or boyfriend who did not support the treatment will certainly be angry if a complication occurs. However, this particular relationship is between the patient and her companion. The fact that her husband is upset is not your responsibility. Her reaction may make your care more challenging, and you should be aware of the situation; communication with both the husband and the wife may be necessary as the complication is healing. Remember, anger is sometimes motivated by fear.

Physical Healing

Healing a complication can be slow and arduous. Patience is required on the part of the clinician, physician, and patient. The most common complication seen in the medical spa is a scar, followed by infections and eye damage. A protocol in your facility should be in place to manage each of these injuries. Follow the protocol to the letter.

Emotional Healing

Emotional healing is just as important as is the physical healing. As stated earlier, the patient must communicate his or her feelings in a safe and trusting environment. Allowing the patient to go through a grieving process is important. Many variables contribute to the patient's emotions during a complication. Patients often feel as though they were too vain, or they should not have spent the money. These feeling are complicated by the fact that they came to your facility to look better, and now they have a scar, creating a great deal of sad and mixed up feelings. Do your best to help the patient get through the grieving process. If you do not feel qualified, then ask a team member who is qualified to help you.

SIDE EFFECTS

A side effect can happen with medications or treatments. However, side effects are most often related to medications. In the case of treatment side effects, rashes or hives from a peel or facial could be considered possible. In reality, the peel solution, mask, or cream used in a treatment causes the problem. The major distinction between a side effect and a complication is that a side effect is not the result of an untoward event but rather the patient's response to the drug or cream used in the treatment. It is possible that, under the same circumstances, the event will happen again. Interestingly, the words *side effects* are rarely if ever used to describe events such as rashes or hives. In fact, most clinicians would consider this reaction a complication. However, rashes or hives are side effects of the topical medication. For example, we would not consider nausea after anesthesia a complication; it is simply a side effect of medications. In the same way, rashes and hives should also be considered side effects of medications or creams in the medical spa. Consents for treatment should reflect the possibility of side effects, and the possibilities should be discussed before treatment.

Clinician Response to Side Effects of Treatment

A clinician's response to side effects will usually coincide with his or her level of experience. Newer clinicians will usually be scared because they have a tendency to assume blame. When a patient sees that you are scared, he or she can easily detect it and, as such, also become scared. Obviously, scaring patients is not in anyone's best interest. If you should become worried, seek out a second opinion, or otherwise follow the documented protocol of the clinic or spa in which you are employed. Similarly, assuming blame is an equally inappropriate response. Patients will not understand the random nature of side effects. They will attach themselves to the notion that it is your fault, or they may deem the side effect as a complication caused by error, or both.

More experienced clinicians will have various reactions as well. On one end of the spectrum, experienced clinicians will have an appropriate response. They have informed their patients of the possibility and react accordingly when the side effect occurs. Experienced clinicians have seen or have heard of the reaction, and therefore their experience equips them to behave in a manner that is best for their patients. On the other hand, some experienced clinicians may become lackadaisical with regard to side effects, ignore them, or take matters into their own hands. The end result of doing so is never positive.

The best response to a side effect is to address the possibility in advance of the treatment and to follow the procedure prescribed by the clinic or spa for which you work. Knowing who should examine the patient and treat the side effects will minimize the damage and restore the trust of the patient.

Patient Education

As always, patient education is one of the most important aspects of patient care. The more accurate information the patient has, the better prepared they will be for the healing course. Discontinuation of the product is usually all that is necessary to alleviate a side effect. However, the patient should always be examined if the response did not happen in the clinic. The patient should also be told all of the products that will be used during a treatment. This process will help elicit a conversation about possible previous product side effects.

Communication and Side Effects

Practicing fair, honest, and compassionate communication is the one skill that can defuse most situations, and it is true of side effect responses as well. The first thing to do is call the reaction by its proper name: a side effect, not a complication. Proper identification will make all of the difference in the world. Everyone understands what a side effect is, but giving the situation clarity and meaning is up to you.

Patient Responses to Side Effects of Treatment

As you know, side effects of treatment are events that are unanticipated, random occurrences that are inconsistent with the expected outcomes of a given treatment. Patients often forget about the side effects, which were ideally discussed during the consultation. Assuming that side effects had been discussed, the patient's normal response to side effects will range from disappointment to fear. The patient's response, as mentioned, will depend greatly on your response to the side effect. Managing the patient's response to side effects will also depend greatly on *your* response to the side effect. This task is accomplished by the degree to which you follow the procedures outlined by the clinic or spa for which you work, as well as your working knowledge. Side effects can sometimes be challenging to evaluate and may require the help of your clinic nurse or physician.

CONSEQUENCES OF TREATMENT

Similar to a complication, a treatment consequence is a known and possible reaction. For example, swelling and bruising are treatment consequences of dermal fillers. In other words, although one would prefer that the event did not occur, the reaction is not unexpected. As previously mentioned, "rug burns" are a treatment consequence of peels, particularly glycolic peels. Some clinicians might mix up the concept of treatment consequences and side effects, but they are two different situations, as you now know. Side effects are not predictable. In many ways, treatment consequences are the easiest problems to manage. Patients are often prepared for them because they are not uncommon. Treatment consequences are involved in the question that you get from the patient before treatment: "What will I look like?" The answer to this question defines a treatment consequence.

Clinician Responses to Consequences of Treatment

The clinician's response to treatment consequences should be minimal. You should be able to anticipate the reaction, and therefore so should the patient. To this effect, the best tool that a clinician can use to manage consequences is patient preparation. Informing patients of the expected consequences, reminding them as they sign the consent form, will minimize the surprise that will invariably create a trust issue between you and your patients.

Patient Education

As in all situations, not enough can be said about patient education. Given that treatment consequences are anticipated, the patient should be made aware before treatment begins. In other words, a direct conversation is necessary that will remind the patient of the possible treatment responses: bruising, swelling, redness, rug burns, peeling, or dry skin, to name a few.

Communication and Consequences

Educating the patient before the treatment begins is important. Then, communication and treatment consequences become simple reassurance procedures for the clinician. In other words, yes, the bruising will resolve; yes, redness will improve; no, the rug burn will not leave a scar. The downfall for the clinician is that the responses can be fairly routine to you, but they are not necessarily routine for the patient. Do not disregard the patient's questions or concerns. If the clinician does not respond to the patient in a compassionate and timely fashion, the relationship will show strain.

Patient Responses to Consequences of Treatment

Patients are often so excited about treatments or so familiar with treatments that they often forget about the concepts of treatment consequences and move on to the idea of results. This tendency is fine most of the time. However, when the patient has a date, or the peeling interferes with, for example, a woman's ability to apply makeup, things can change.

Therefore your responsibility immediately after the treatment is to remind the patient of the possible treatment consequences. Written material is the best tool for this task. The best written material is customized by treatment and by day. For example, "On the day of treatment your skin will appear...." "The day after treatment your skin will appear...." Literature that is specifically directed continues the patient educational process and decreases the opportunity for problems and disappointment.

Physical Healing

Physical healing for consequences of treatment usually occurs during the recovery period specific to the treatment, meaning that 3 to 5 days are needed to heal from a certain treatment which takes into consideration the consequences that are almost certain to occur. Consequences that take longer may, in fact, be complications and should be examined to ensure proper recovery.

▶ ▷ ▷ TOP TEN TIPS TO TAKE TO THE CLINIC

1. Know the difference between complications and consequences of treatment.
2. Do not treat consequences as if they are complications.
3. Patient education is an important component of a successful treatment.
4. Be familiar with common patient responses to treatment consequences.
5. Be familiar with common patient responses to complications.
6. Do not be discouraged if the patient does not want you to care for them any longer.
7. Understand and respect the patient's feelings of anger, regret, and embarrassment.
8. Refine and improve your communication skills.
9. Practice self-awareness.
10. Recognize the difference between physical healing and emotional healing.

CHAPTER REVIEW QUESTIONS

1. What are complications?
2. What are treatment consequences?
3. What are side effects?
4. How is communication helpful in a difficult situation?
5. What are the patient's common responses to a complication?

BIBLIOGRAPHY

Thomas, C. L. (Ed.). (1997). *Taber's cyclopedia medical dictionary* (Vol. 18). Philadelphia: F. A. Davis.

CHAPTER REFERENCES

1. Thomas, C. L. (Ed.). (1997). *Taber's cyclopedia medical dictionary* (Vol. 18). Philadelphia: F. A. Davis.
2. Life Impact. (2005, May 27). *Emotional intelligence (EQ)*. [Online]. Available: http://www.lifeimpact.co.nz

Characteristics of the Best Clinical Experience

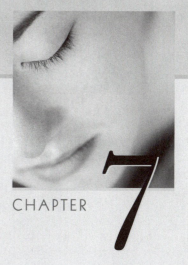

KEY TERMS

fad   Thermage®   trends
radio frequency   treatment history

CHAPTER 7

LEARNING OBJECTIVES

After completing this chapter you should be able to:

1. Identify three characteristics that help create an optimal outcome for the patient.
2. Discuss the importance of training in the optimal outcome.
3. Identify three reasons why a positive attitude will contribute to an optimal outcome for the patient.
4. Discuss the importance of the spa environment.

INTRODUCTION

In earlier chapters, we discussed different components that contribute to an optimal outcome. We learned the core concepts of society and communication and how they contribute to the clinical concepts of consultations, treatment plans, and treatments themselves. Providing an optimal outcome can be expanded to all aspects of the clinical environment. From the choice of equipment to the products in stock, many steps can be made to provide the patient with the best result and a superior outcome. In this chapter, we will discuss some of the more controllable aspects that can contribute to or, in some instances, detract from an optimal outcome. Among these aspects are training, technology, location, and style.

■ TRAINING

Aside from your current studies, a thorough training and a regular continuing-education program will pay for themselves in the long run. Training gives way to good patient care and excellent results. After years on the job, many clinicians become complacent, sighting that they have done treatments so many times, they can "do it in their sleep." This statement might be acceptable if technology, information, and treatments remained fixed. In reality, these processes constantly evolve. As a student of aesthetics, your homework will go on long after you have completed your education. The most successful clinicians will be the ones who will always be on the lookout for new information or innovations that will reap positive results for their client base and, as such, themselves. Some of the best places to acquire training or continuing education can be an in-house program at your clinic, by way of the Internet, or at shows or trade industry conferences. That said, training is not as simple as it once was; our industry is more complex. More products, more treatments, and more technology have become available. Plus, rarely does a school or manufacturer provide unbiased, comprehensive training to benefit the clinician. What is a clinician to do? Read, read, and read some more, and analyze what you read. Network with other clinicians in your industry, use Web chat rooms, talk with colleagues, and write in a diary or journal. Subscribe to trade industry magazines and newsletters. Collect information as often as possible, sift through it, keep the good stuff, and throw away the bad. As you continue to advance your sphere of knowledge, you will become more of an asset to yourself and your employer, which will provide you with job security. Similarly, your patients will easily recognize your know-how and also be comforted by your aptitude for your profession. The same cannot be said for the employee who does not take an active role in the training or continuing-education process. People who are not serious about their training regimens will yield negative results for their patients, as well as the clinic.

■ TECHNOLOGY

Technology is ever changing. New products and treatments that are making their debut on the market right now may be outdated and out of fashion tomorrow. Because of this constant fluctuation, keeping up with technologic advances in the aesthetics industry will require tenacity and reason. Even though you will be confronted with an ever-changing buffet of treatment options to learn, using some industry savvy will help sort out the **trends** and **fad**. Doing so will make the most efficient use of your time and resources, enabling you to consider only the technologic advances that will be most cost effective over the long run.

Technology drives our industry by putting additional choices in front of patients. Savvy patients will also be on the lookout for new innovations that will further their goals. At times, some patients will ask you for your opinion or information about new treatments. This instance is when keeping up with innovation comes in handy. If you have knowledge about the treatment, you can answer the patient's questions. Otherwise, consider how you might feel if your patients know more about what is on the marketplace than you do.

Having general unbiased knowledge of the newest technologies will help guide patients. For example, **Thermage**® or the newest treatments using **radio frequency** (RF) may be demanded by patients, but these new technologies have not been available long enough to provide a **treatment history**. Technology requires training, but it also requires a treatment history. "How do you know that clients will embrace next year the technology you buy today?" How do you know if the technology that they embrace will provide and sustain the results that are alleged?

Furthermore, states are becoming strict about the registration and use of qualified and approved equipment in the salon and spa. The National Coalition of Esthetic & Related Associations (NCEA) has developed a registration form and process for equipment manufacturers that allow for easy state registration. If you are wondering about the qualifications of a piece of equipment, the NCEA should have the answer. You can contact the NCEA at the following web site: http://www.ncea.tv

trends
A prevailing tendency.

fad
A temporary fashion or manner of conduct.

Thermage®
A noninvasion radio-frequency technology to improve facial appearance.

radio frequency
A frequency of transmitting radio waves.

treatment history
A period that is long enough to assess results, usually 2 years.

All of that said, technology and its results are the wave of the future. It builds business, gives the clinician new tools, and improves the results for the patients.

■ TRENDS VERSUS FADS

Trends and fads are pervasive in our pop-culture society. In many instances, the words are used interchangeably and are thus confusing. Someone wearing only the latest fashions might be called "trendy," for example. In fact, saying that the person is more into fads than he or she is into trends is probably more accurate. What is the difference between a trend and a fad?

Fads ebb and flow with greater speed compared with trends. The only basis for something to be a fad is that it gains popularity with a relatively small group of people, usually a subculture. A fad can remain a fad for a long time before it either fades or makes its way into the mainstream. Once a fad emerges in the mainstream, it becomes a trend. A trend is a course of prevailing tendencies over time and space. It is the result of a variety of indicators over a period, which suggests a general directional flow ideology. For example, a trend in aesthetics might be a preference for hyaluronic acid over bovine collagen for dermal fillers. If over a wide swath of territory, bovine collagen is on the decrease, and hyaluronic acid is equally increasing, you can see where the basis for the trend is derived.

Nonetheless, patients who prefer the tried and true exist, and they are unwilling to move with the newest trends. What causes certain people to move with the masses and others to stay behind? This question, of course, is one for the sociologist to answer. However, in the aesthetics world, the brief answer might be found in the comfort of results and safety and of clinician know-how.

■ SERVICES

As clinicians, we sell services and products. However, we also sell image and a modicum of luxurious escape. How do you put it all together and stay within the concept that you have developed for yourself? Some basics that are still the crux to a successful outcome should be considered, no matter what services, product, or spa you happen to offer. These basics include location, environment (decorating, cleanliness, color, and so forth), the products, and the services that are offered.

In the service category, the following questions should be considered. Which services should be offered, and why? Which services are most profitable, and why? Which services work well together, and why? The next factor to consider is the physical space. How big will the spa be, and why? What will be the scheme of the spa? How will retail products be sold? Finally, where is the best location?

Although these questions appear to be merely business questions on the surface, in reality, we are dealing with questions that, in the end, will create either a positive outcome or a potentially negative experience for the patient. All aspects should be considered potential opportunities to improve patient outcome.

ENVIRONMENT AND LOCATION

Prevailing theory suggests that the success of a retail business depends on three things: location, location, and location. However, before selecting a location, you have to decide *what you are;* a luxury day spa would not work in a medical office building, but a medical spa might work fine in this same location.

Additionally, you need to know your competition in the area. If you are a luxury spa, having an elegant address will enhance the overall image of the business. In aesthetics, an aesthetically pleasing environment is obviously crucial to your success.

The environment of the spa is as much a component of the branding as are services, products, brochures, and employees. Patients who are looking for a medical spa expect a lifestyle experience. Although the majority of Americans do not believe that a spa experience is a long-term approach to wellness or healing, a core group of people believes that going to a spa is an integral part of their health routine.[1] This concept is especially true for people who frequent a medical spa. A focus on wellness and skin care are important to this small group of *spa-goers.*

Criteria Used to Evaluate Equipment

- Safety certification (Underwriters Laboratory or Canadian Standard Association)
- U.S. Food and Drug Administration's "Intended Use Statement"
- The manufacturer's "Intended Use Statement"
- Product liability insurance
- Will your malpractice insurance cover the procedures you intend to perform with this equipment?
- Colleagues' evaluations and recommendations

A debate exists as to the best location for medical spas. Different clinics have attempted many different types of locations, from strip malls to medical office buildings. However, the debate rages on as industry standards are defined. Some people might argue that a hospital or medical plaza is best. This location facilitates the notion that more advanced or *medicinal* treatments are offered. Additionally, this location makes collaborating with physicians or nurses, who are more likely to be nearby, easier. However, this location may be intimidating to patients who might be fearful. Regardless of where the office is situated, a professional appearance, the responsibility of being a medical facility, and image should be considered. The environment within the clinic should be consistent with both the medical side (more clinical and private) and the spa side (luxurious and pleasant).

The environment should invite and accommodate the needs of the consumer. This concept should be reflected in all aspects, from the decor to the treatments themselves. Interior design and ritual and innovative marketing are keys to driving loyalty with clients to the aesthetic business. The environment should be gender neutral and refined. It should appeal to men and women, as well as the newest consumers: children.

■ PRODUCTS

Products are an important revenue source for all spas. Product displays should be pleasant looking, and they should be clean and dust free. They should be selected in conjunction with the services that are being offered. Products should also coincide with the goals of the client. If clients come to the spa for relaxation and pampering, products should be selected that will offer the client the opportunity to take some pampering home with them.

Given that the menu of treatment options are more varied and often advanced at a medical spa, the skin-care products should reflect the

---

Criteria Used to Evaluate Products

- Does it support the treatments provided at the spa?
- Are the vendors friendly and accommodative?
- Do the ingredients fit with the spa philosophies?
- Are the products fairly priced and provide a reasonable markup?
- Is the manufacturer innovative and creative?

advanced nature of these treatments. Most notably different in the medical spa product line are prescriptions.

Because of the use of prescriptions, patients and regulators expect the products to be effective. Therefore these same items will also be under more scrutiny, as will the clinician.

■ STAFFING

Every spa, and every business for that matter, struggles with getting and keeping *good help*. Optimal outcomes depend on expert staff. High turnover rates are costly for a clinic. Patients will become uncomfortable when too many clinicians become involved in what many would deem an *uncomfortable* or *private* situation. Similarly, new or inexperienced staff members are more likely to make mistakes, which will certainly affect the bottom line.

Positive Attitudes

Positive attitudes and good customer service make a difference to the success of any business but in personal services especially. Some people might argue that nothing can be more important.

Consider your own retail experiences. Suppose you encounter a clerk who is angry, and his or her body language says so. The clerk throws down your change and waits for you to leave. Next, imagine you are in the shop of a high-end clothier. You are waiting for assistance, but the assistants are preoccupied with their conversation with one another. These instances are two different situations with a similar outcome. Almost certainly, you left the establishment discouraged, questioning whether you should return again. The same experience is likely to occur if you project the same negativity to your clients. Good customer service and a pleasant disposition will make the patient want to come back to your facility every time.

Given that all types of spas are about regenerating the spirit, as well as improving appearance, a bad attitude will have greater consequences than if you worked as a clerk or at the clothier. Positive attitudes create optimal outcomes; both clients and staff will benefit from as much.

Teamwork

Just as a positive attitude will create an optimal outcome, the same applies to teamwork. Teamwork is important because it will provide the patient with the best outcome. Similarly, a patient who notices a team working in cohesion is likely to give his or her trust over to the team.

To this avail, teamwork helps the spa run more efficiently and improves the rhythm of the spa.

Conclusion

Optimal outcomes are, in part, a result of the spa experience: the location, the environment, and the concepts of training, a positive attitude, and teamwork. We would be remiss if we did not again mention the importance of technology.

Optimal outcomes is a complex concept, without clarity to the multiple levels, that can easily be interpreted as simply that which applies to the treatment itself when, in fact, it is far more complex.

TOP TEN TIPS TO TAKE TO THE CLINIC

1. Choosing the service menu will define the type of spa.
2. Quality staffing is an important component of positive patient outcome.
3. Rhythmic teamwork positively contributes to positive patient outcome.
4. Branding helps direct the client to the proper spa for his or her treatments.
5. Knowing the difference between a trend and a fad will help ensure a positive outcome.
6. Technology is the wave of the future.
7. Teams are similar to small societies, with all the inherent problems and benefits.
8. Products can extend the spa experience.
9. The spa environment can affect the quality of the patient outcome.
10. Choose your equipment for the spa carefully.

CHAPTER REVIEW QUESTIONS

1. How does the environment of the spa influence the outcome of the experience?
2. How are medical spas different from other types of spas?
3. How does a positive attitude on the part of the staff influence the patient outcome?
4. How do take-home products expand the spa experience?
5. How does branding affect the quality of the spa outcome?

BIBLIOGRAPHY

Brown, A. (2005, January 25). *Top ten spa trends.* [Online]. Available: www.spas.about.com

International SPA Association. (2004, November). *Consumer trends report: Executive summary.* [Online]. Available: http://www.experienceispa. com

CHAPTER REFERENCE

1. International SPA Association. (2004, November). *Consumer trends report: Executive summary.* [Online]. Available: http://www. experienceispa.com

Getting the Most Out of the Top Five Aesthetic Procedures

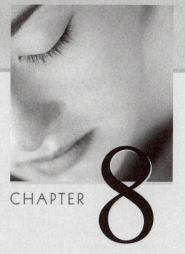

CHAPTER 8

KEY TERMS

collagen
contraindications
dermabrasion
glycosaminoglycans
granulomas

ground substance
indications
magnetic resonance
    imaging
necrosis

nonsurgical aesthetic
    skin care
phenol
Propionibacterium acnes
trichloroacetic acid

LEARNING OBJECTIVES

After completing this chapter you should be able to:

1. Discuss the benefits of aesthetics treatments.
2. Discuss the importance of patient education.
3. Define pretreatment, and discuss the importance of this step.
4. Discuss the steps of treatment follow-up.

INTRODUCTION

Lines, wrinkles, and sagging skin were once considered as irreversible consequences of the aging process. Prior generations grudgingly accepted their right of passage into the golden years. Some people wore their lines proudly as a testament to their survival through war, depression, and oppression. Today, the opposite is true; the signs of aging are considered unwarranted and unwanted. As the baby boomers pass into their own golden years, they have been responsible for the creation of a multi-billion dollar industry we call **nonsurgical aesthetic skin care.** Wanting to sustain a youthful appearance, these baby boomers and the generations that follow them have forced our industry to develop products and services to meet their needs.

One needs to look only as far as reality television to see that our society is obsessed with looking better. People subject themselves to numerous surgical procedures to transform, sometimes radically, the way they look. Although this measure is extreme, everyone has a desire to improve themselves and enhance their appearance. Whether we like it or not, our society is "looks oriented," rewarding younger, more attractive people. Good-looking people seem to land better jobs, usually making more money. They seem to have more friends and are welcomed more in social situations. With so much on the line, how do patients gain the most benefits from the procedures they have selected?

For the aesthetician, this tendency means finding the best ways to ensure that the patient experience provides them with not only good results, but also a positive outcome. In this chapter, we will review some of the more common treatments, while offering advice that will help maximize the clinical experience for all parties involved.

nonsurgical aesthetic skin care
Any noninvasive procedure that is intended to improve overall skin health and appearance.

▪ BENEFITS OF AESTHETIC TREATMENTS

The benefits of aesthetic treatments can be numerous and do not apply just to the skin or cosmetic surgery. Consider cosmetic dental procedures and hair cutting and coloring. The benefits that a patient gains include an improved appearance, an increase in self-esteem, and a positive experience.

In the context of aesthetics, a positive experience is the single most important thing that will motivate the patient to return for more treatments or refer others for a similar experience.

Positive experiences are promoted when the patient is educated and has appropriate pretreatment, treatment education, and posttreatment care. When the clinician has a variety of technology apparatus from which to choose, he or she must understand the technology and be capable of using the technology. Technology does not always mean equipment, lasers, radio frequency, or microdermabrasion, but can also mean product technology or procedural advances as well.

Bearing all of these variables in mind, let us have a look at some of the most important tactics that provide an optimal patient outcome.

Technical Aspects that Render an Optimal Outcome

As we discussed earlier, the clinician should understand all the technology available to him or her to make the right decision for the patient and his or her problems. This concept requires the clinician to invest time in researching and understanding new technologies as they come into the marketplace.

The clinician should be capable in using the technology in question to provide the intended outcome. The intended outcome may be simply seeking information, in which case, knowing what you are talking about will virtually ensure an optimal outcome. However, when performing a new procedure, adequate training and information combined are necessary.

If training is required, contacting the manufacturer, as well as practice, are important before treating patients.

Patient Education

Education promotes a positive experience for clients. Not only will they feel good about newfound knowledge, but they can also better understand their requirements and necessity of home-care programs and treatments. Knowledge is power. The more patients know, the more cooperative they will be. Additionally, they will understand the possibilities and limitations of the treatments.

Imparting the information in a clear, understandable fashion will help achieve an optimal level of understanding. The clinician has to know what material is needed to educate the patient; if you do not know the information, you cannot be effective for the patient. This concept means separating the wheat from the chafe, so to speak. Knowing what is important and what is not important will make understanding the material and retaining the material easier for the patient.

Pretreatment

One of the most valuable pieces of information that the patient needs to understand is the pretreatment or home-care requirements to which they must adhere. The time when the patient is preparing for the treatment, usually at home, is just as important to the outcome as are the treatments that you will be providing. This concept is important and requires attention. As we mentioned, just because you tell patients the information does not mean they are listening. Speak clearly, and engage patients. Repeat information if necessary, and answer any questions. Finally, write it down for patients so they have something to which to refer when they get home. Most importantly, tell patients that adherence is crucial to the outcome. This final point is often the "X" factor; therefore imparting this information early and often will be the responsibility of the clinician. Patients need to understand the purpose.

Follow-Up

After treatment, while the patient is healing, support and further education will be required. Sometimes, even though they were forewarned, patients will be shocked by their appearance following certain treatments, such as advanced peels. This time can be difficult for patients, and the clinician should have patience. Place a call to these patients, daily if needed. Reassure them that their discomfort and unattractive appearance is a means to an end. Ask questions, and listen to patients' concerns. Be on the lookout for complications or side effects. During healing, patients can become depressed, regretful, or disappointed. If this is the case, ensuring that patients remember the steps of the healing process is important. Your contact with a patient after treatment will console, inspire, and remind the patient of the mutual goals toward which you are working.

■ MICRODERMABRASION

With microdermabrasion treatment, variations in the techniques used, the machine selected, the clinician, and the condition of the skin combine to affect the result. The pros and cons of crystal type, vacuum settings, or positive pressure, as well as clinical and home-care products, create fodder for continued debate. This section will take on the controversies of microdermabrasion technology, techniques, and the result, much of which is directly related to patient selection, clinician training, and experience.

Our objective is to quiet this discussion, focusing our attention on the patient and potential result and creating an optimal microdermabrasion experience for the patient. To do so requires guidelines that reduce, as much as possible, the variability found in microdermabrasion treatments. Within this section, we will discuss subjects that will help simplify and demystify microdermabrasion and direct the clinician to a predictable outcome.

The idea of sanding the skin to improve its appearance is a long-standing technique used by plastic surgeons and cosmetic dermatologists. Whether the physician is using a small wire brush or pieces of actual sandpaper to abrade the skin in combination with chemical peeling, surgeons have had success "sanding" the skin to improve its appearance. Although microdermabrasion is not a surgical resurfacing tool, it has its origins in surgical resurfacing procedures such as **dermabrasion.** Microdermabrasion and dermabrasion have one overriding similarity in that both procedures start from the premise that sanding the skin will improve its appearance. Obviously, the depth of the procedures and the number of treatments are the factors that significantly differ.

Similar to dermabrasion, microdermabrasion also sands the skin, but the apparatus (crystals versus wire brush or sandpaper) is different, and the depth is more superficial, more like polishing. Microdermabrasion also has much broader application, addressing fine lines, dyschromias, texture issues, acne scarring, small scars, and solar keratosis.

Patient Selection

Not all skin types or skin problems are appropriate for microdermabrasion. Carefully selecting the candidates is the clinician's responsibility, ensuring that the particular skin condition can be improved or solved by the treatment. This measure is the first step to ensure that the patient has a predictable result and an acceptable outcome. **Indications** and **contraindications** can sometimes overlap, producing a challenging decision for the clinician. To overcome this dilemma, the clinician must take the consultation process seriously, listening to the patient carefully and identifying the primary problem. Based on predetermined indications and contraindications, the problem can then be evaluated. Using conservative judgment is always the best approach; but sometimes our enthusiasm to help a patient's skin will cloud our judgment. Using the indications and contraindications as a tool in the evaluation process will help avoid poor judgment and subsequent poor outcomes.

Dermabrasion is a rarely used skin-resurfacing technique developed in the early 1900s. The procedure uses a small wire brush or diamond-coated wheel to "sand" the skin. The wheel turns quickly, producing injury to the skin at the papillary dermis and sometimes deeper.

dermabrasion
Predecessor to microdermabrasion that used a wire brush or a diamond-coated wheel to resurface the skin from the papillary dermal level.

indications
Any sign or circumstance indicating that a particular treatment is appropriate or warranted.

contraindications
Any sign or symptom indicating that a particular treatment, which would otherwise be advisable, would be inappropriate.

Patient Education

Medical skin care has always ascribed to the notion that pretreatment is the foundation to a favorable outcome. Even in the "old days," Retin A® and hydroquinone were considered an important step before a **phenol** or **trichloroacetic acid** peel. The complexity of pretreatment and the understanding of its necessity are now quite advanced. Pretreatment before surgical or nonsurgical procedures with an advanced regimented home-care routine is now considered the standard of care. Many clients who will come to your office will be skeptical of medical skin-care programs. Their body language and attitude says, "Prove it." These clients may be devotees of a particular brand of product, or they may be determined to stick with plain *soap and water*. The basis of their skepticism is the result of years of product purchases, with limited or no results. Regardless of their product dedication, these patients still have hopes for improvement, no matter how hidden these hopes may be. A thorough explanation of the regimen and its importance is necessary to educate the client that the changes and expense are justified. Obviously, education will also play into our ability to provide a predictable outcome and hence a quality experience.

■ PEELS

Every day, our skin is undergoing the normal process of sloughing older dead skin cells. In place of these dead cells, newer cells have traveled up through the layers of skin. They will replace the dead cells and ultimately suffer the same fate. However, as we get older, the time required for the older cells to slough off increases. This fact means that the older cells stay in place longer, causing our skin to appear dull and aged.

Chemical peels accelerate this process in three different ways. First, resurfacing the stratum corneum stimulates epidermal growth, which makes the epidermis thicken. Second, chemical peels cause **necrosis,** or destruction of damaged skin. Ideally, the damaged or dyschromatic skin will be replaced with healthier, normalized tissue by means of the skin's wound-healing processes. Finally, deeper peels will induce the production of new **collagen** and **ground substance** within the dermis.

Chemical peels are exactly as they sound: using agents to peel the outermost layer or layers of skin, allowing newer and healthier skin to present itself. Peels can be an individual procedure or a single step in a multifaceted treatment. However, the types of peels, as well as peel depths, are numerous. Some of the deeper peels can cause serious injury, more so than most other treatments that an aesthetician will perform for patients. Deep peels are the ones with the greatest amount of success

phenol
A highly corrosive acid used in peel solutions, which dissolves cells to make room for newer and healthier ones.

trichloroacetic acid
A chemical used in peel solutions that dissolve aging cells to make room for newer, healthier ones.

necrosis
The death of cells when tissue is deprived of blood supply.

collagen
An insoluble protein found in connective tissues. Particularly, type I collagen forms a network in the epidermis, and it is credited with providing skin with its tensile strength and firmness.

ground substance
A substance that consists mainly of glycosaminoglycans (hyaluronic acid, chondroitin sulfate, and dermatan sulfate) involved in maintenance and repair of dermis.

and potential for complications. A thorough understanding of chemical peels is vital to your success as an aesthetician.

Chemical peels have an expansive appeal with both young and old individuals. With many positive attributes to recommend it, chemical peels are the preferred treatment for many signs of aging, including dyschromias and fine lines. However, these results do not come without risks. Depending on the particular peel, the downtime can be significant in addition to the risk of complications such as infection and scarring.

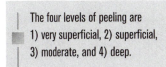

The four levels of peeling are 1) very superficial, 2) superficial, 3) moderate, and 4) deep.

Patient Selection

The principles that are to be taken into consideration before peeling the skin are the skin condition, the skin type, the aging factor, and the patient's general health. These important variables assist the clinician in selecting the proper candidates for peel treatment, as well as the appropriate solution to meet everyone's goal. This process is, of course, the groundwork for our optimal outcome. The skin condition includes not only the five definitive categorizations with which we are familiar (i.e., dry, oily or acne prone, sensitive, combination), but also skin problems. Additional descriptors of skin problems are necessary, that is to say, dyschromias, wrinkles, aging, and acne. This additional descriptor will assist us in determining possible indications and contraindications for the peel.

Remember, indications and contraindications are conditions that determine whether a treatment is appropriate or inappropriate. As you consider a patient for treatment, you must determine whether the skin conditions you wish to treat will be affected by the peel treatment you choose or, for that matter, by peeling at all. Just as important is the skin type. A Fitzpatrick skin typing analysis must be done to determine whether the patient is likely to have a positive treatment outcome. Similarly, an aging analysis must be determined. The skin typing and age analysis exercise should answer the following questions: "Will the skin have a propensity for hyperpigmentation?" "Will the skin peel evenly?" "What chemical will be necessary to achieve the result?" "Will the skin actually improve?" Last, and not to be disregarded, is the patient's health status. Unlike a simple microdermabrasion treatment, chemical peels are more likely to be affected by the patient's health status. Because the chemical peel is a *controlled burn*, the clinician must understand the impact of a burn on the body.

Patient Education

Chemical peeling has many benefits that cannot be duplicated by other spa or clinical treatments. Among these benefits are increasing the

glycosaminoglycans
Polysaccharide chains, most
prominent in the dermis, that bind
with water, smoothing and softening
the surface from below.

To avoid disappointment, a full
consultation with the patient is
necessary. This consultation
should include a discussion of
desired results, downtime, health
status, and the patient's current
skin-care program. The clinician
should also evaluate the indications for peeling at this time.

glycosaminoglycans in the ground substance of the skin, thickening the epidermis, and increasing collagen remodeling in the dermis. These improvements result in healthier skin that appears more vibrant and youthful. The best responses to chemical peeling are achieved when the patient's objectives, the peel solution, the skin indications, and the clinician's ability all coincide. The patient's objectives should be ascertained at the initial consultation or at a peel consultation. Included in this discussion should be the patient's desired end result, the amount of downtime available, and the health status. The clinician should also evaluate whether the patient will be able to follow the postcare instructions. Chemical peels can be ugly in the healing process, and some patients cannot emotionally tolerate their appearance. Ascertaining whether the patient is a good *emotional* candidate is also important. Other information that is collected includes the indications and contraindications. This information will drive some of the decision about the peel solution selection. Remember, the depth of the peel is directly related to the end result. Therefore, if you are trying to remedy deeper rhytids, a deeper peel is in order. On the other hand, if you are trying to resolve fine lines, lighter repetitive peeling will work fine.

The clinician must understand, before treatment begins, what a peel can do and what a peel cannot do. This level of clarity will alleviate misunderstandings with the patient and frustration on the part of the clinician. This situation alone is cause for a poor outcome, regardless of the actual peel result. Among the indications for light chemical peeling are dyschromias, rough textures, fine lines, and acne grades 1 and 2. Indications for medium peeling are rhytids, dyschromias, and rough textures. Patients with loose skin and deeper lines (who do not choose a facial surgery) will benefit from a deep phenol peel.

▪ FACIALS

In the past, facials have often been viewed as a luxury available only to women of wealth and leisure, but this is no longer true. Facials, in fact, have become a critical part of a good skin-care program, medical or otherwise. Facials not only clean and stimulate the skin, but the process itself also allows for relaxation, a much-needed break in today's busy world.

Facials come in all shapes and sizes. European steam facials are the most recognized, but many other types of facials appropriate for the skin are available, including some facial fads that are just plain fun. Many types of common facials are available, including, but not limited to, hydrating facial, acne facial, vitamin C facial, and American (nonsteam) facial. In the category of fads, we have fruit facials or chocolate facials.

Performing a facial involves a few basics steps: cleansing, skin analysis, exfoliation, massage, extraction of blackheads and other impurities, and application of products targeted to the skin type (dry, oily, combination, sensitive, and mature). A hand and foot massage is sometimes given while the masque is drying. Facials can also involve other elements such as aromatherapy (using essential oils to soothe, relax, or energize the patient), glycolic acid treatments (helping to refine skin), a scalp massage, or applying herbs or concoctions that are supposed to make the skin look better.

Patient Selection

Choosing ideal candidates for facials is fairly cut and dried. Generally, all patients are candidates for facials, especially those who have other treatments, such as microdermabrasion, on a monthly basis. Sensitive skin should be monitored but is never excluded from a monthly facial. Patients with sensitive skin are sometimes prone to irritation, and these patients should be notified of this reaction. Once again, communication and education are the keys to an optimal outcome.

During the procedure, the clinician should be gentle and prepare the patient for each step of the process. If products are warm or cold, warning the patient can make for a more enjoyable experience. Remember, communicate with the patient. Ask about your touch, the temperature of the room, the comfort of the bed, and other elements that will make the experience more enjoyable.

Patient Education

Clients who are receiving facials can be doing so either in preparation for another treatment or solely by itself. These patients are usually aiming to achieve a certain level of relaxation. However, clients who are getting only a facial may be prone to heightened expectations. As with any other procedure, pinpointing the exact goal of the patient is to your advantage. If the expectations are unreasonable, reeducation and revision of the expectations is in order.

Be warned that your patient's face will be somewhat red for a day or two after treatment, especially if many extractions occur. Discourage patients from scheduling a facial right before a big event, such as a wedding or high school reunion, especially if this is a first or random facial. On the other hand, regular facials can actually make skin's texture improve and reduce the episodes of breakouts.

Patients who are pregnant, are wearing contacts, or have any allergies or other health concerns will require special attention. Be sure to consult with your clinic physician (if available) if you have any concerns.

■ PERMANENT MAKEUP

Tattooing has been used for centuries by people in all walks of life. Most often, people who receive tattoos do so for aesthetic reasons, others for more personal reasons. One increasingly common type of aesthetic tattooing is permanent makeup. Why would someone choose to have this done? Simply stated, it is easier. For people who are physically inhibited or just plain tired of daily application of temporary makeup, permanent makeup is an ideal solution. For other people, tattooing is an adjunct to cosmetic surgery to simulate natural pigmentation. People who have lost their eyebrows may choose to have eyebrows tattooed on, while people with vitiligo (a lack of pigmentation in areas of the skin) may try tattooing to help recolor the skin.

As the popularity of tattooing and permanent makeup grows, regulatory agencies such as the U.S. Food and Drug Administration have begun taking a closer look at safety. Among the issues under consideration are tattoo removal, adverse reactions to tattoo colors, and complications such as infections that result from tattooing. Also of concern are the pigments themselves and the diluents being used in tattooing: more than 50 different pigments are approved for use in cosmetics but are not approved for injection into the skin. Many pigments used in tattoo inks are not approved for skin contact at all. In fact, some of these pigments are industrial grade, suitable for printer's ink or automobile paint.

Therefore, although permanent makeup is gaining popularity with aging baby boomers, the regulatory issues, pigment safety, and licensure of technicians is in its infancy.

Patient Selection

Recipients of permanent makeup, like facials, come from all walks of life. Women looking for a break from their daily makeup regimes are the usual candidates. However, men and increasingly younger women are also having the procedure done. For many people, permanent makeup gives some patients shelter from the self-consciousness created by defects or disease. For example, people with partial or complete hair loss as a result of chemotherapy or other conditions that cause alopecia (hair loss) can benefit from permanent makeup. Other conditions that result in variations in the skin pigment, such as vitiligo, use permanent makeup successfully. Aside from patients after surgery, many recipients of permanent makeup are people who are vision and motor impaired. For these patients, being able to look good while maintaining a modicum of independence goes a long way (Table 8–1).

Table 8–1 Types of Permanent Cosmetic Procedures

Eyebrows
Eyeliner, top and bottom
Eyelash enhancement
Lip liner
Full lip color
Scar camouflage
Feature reconstruction
Areola restoration or repigmentation
Hair imitation
Skin grafts
Cleft lip, harelip
Beauty marks

Patient Education

When discussing the application of permanent makeup with a patient, as with all procedures, you should discuss the risks associated with the procedure. With permanent makeup, weighing the risks is especially important considering its long-term nature. To that effect, patients must know that permanent makeup is, in fact, permanent. Even considering the advancement in laser removal treatments, removing the pigment may be accomplished only by scarring. The removal process can also be especially risky if permanent makeup has been on or around the eyes.

The other risk that needs to be discussed with potential candidates is the possibility of infection. Unsterile tattooing equipment and needles can transmit infectious diseases such as hepatitis. The risk of infection is the reason the American Association of Blood Banks requires a 1-year wait between getting a tattoo and donating blood. Making sure that all tattooing equipment is clean and sterilized before use is extremely important. Even if the needles are sterilized or have never been used, an important point to understand is that, in some cases, the equipment that holds the needles cannot be sterilized reliably because of its design.

In addition, the person who receives a tattoo must be sure to care for the tattooed area properly during the first week or so after the pigments are injected.

Although allergic reactions to tattoo pigments are rare, when they happen, they may be particularly troublesome because the pigments can be hard to remove. Occasionally, people may develop an allergic reaction to tattoos they have had for years. An example of this is **granulomas,** nodules that may form around material that the body perceives as foreign, which can occur from particles of tattoo pigment.

One rarely known risk associated with permanent makeup, or tattooing in general, is the possibility of swelling or burning in tattooed areas while undergoing **magnetic resonance imaging** (MRI). This reaction is associated with the iron oxides in the pigment and is of concern to technicians operating MRI equipment.

granulomas
A tumor caused by foreign bodies.

magnetic resonance imaging
A noninvasive diagnostic technique that produces computerized images of internal body tissues.

■ TECHNOLOGY-BASED TREATMENTS

Intense pulsed light (IPL) technology improves the appearance of photo-aged skin, removes age spots (sunlight-induced freckles), most benign brown pigments, and redness caused by broken capillaries through a process called photo-rejuvenation. IPL is used for the face and the body. The process is ideal for patients with active lifestyles because the procedure requires no downtime and produces few side effects. The gentle, nonablative treatments use broad-spectrum light to treat the face, chest, neck and hands—virtually anywhere that solar damage shows.

Laser hair removal is increasing in popularity as a way of removing hair, offering unsurpassed results to the greatest variety of patients. Lumenis™ products have led the way in making effective hair removal a mainstay of leading aesthetic practices. With both the LightSheer™ diode lasers and IPL™ systems for hair removal services, physicians are able to offer hair removal that will effectively treat all hair colors and textures, including blonde and gray hair, as well as very fine hair. The newest machines also treat darker skin, without depigmentation or scarring.

Thermage™ is a noninvasive treatment that uses radio frequency to deliver a treatment to the skin. This cutting-edge technology is a noninvasive treatment for the face, targeting rhytids. The treatment will improve the facial contours and collagen in the dermis and is appropriate for all skin types. The device works by heating and cooling the skin without ablation. This deep heat causes the structures of the skin's dermis to remodel into younger, healthier skin.

ClearLight™ is a new method to treat acne. From a medical standpoint, acne is not life threatening and, as such, receives only moderate attention in the advanced-technology category. However, acne is a widespread and embarrassing condition. It can produce lifelong scars, both physically and emotionally. As we know, acne typically begins in adolescence and can continue well into adulthood. Associated with enlarged and obstructed sebaceous glands, the skin becomes inflamed and exhibits pustules and papules. The abnormal bacteria usually associated with acne are **Propionibacterium acnes** *(P. acnes)*. The newest technology available to treat acne is a blue light, trade name ClearLight™. The ClearLight™ system uses a high-intensity, enhanced, narrow-band light source (405 to 420 nm) to destroy *P. acnes* bacteria. Patients are treated in the clinic on a regular basis to great success.

Polaris Elos™ is a bipolar radio-frequency system. This combined energy creates predictable outcomes with lower energy levels, ensuring patient comfort and superior results. This machine is multifunctional and can be used for wrinkle treatment, leg vein resolution, hair removal, and photo-rejuvenation.

Propionibacterium acnes
Bacteria that cause a tumor produced when the body fails to destroy foreign body product or mycobacteria.

Patient Selection

Success with advanced high technology depends on proper patient selection, clinician knowledge, advanced patient education, and realistic expectations for both clinician and patient. Therefore proper analysis of patients' ability to understand and follow instructions will be important to the final outcome. A list of criteria for patient selection should be available to guide the clinician in the decision-making process.

Patient Education

As with other procedures, patient education is among the most important keys to a positive and optimal outcome. The educational process will be more involved when the clinician is dealing with technology and the potential risks, as well as results.

Conclusion

Optimal outcomes in each procedure may be specific to the procedure, but general guidelines help the clinician ensure success. These guidelines include patient selection, patient education, and understanding the procedure, including its possibilities and limitations.

▶ ⟩ ⟩ TOP TEN TIPS TO TAKE TO THE CLINIC

1. Understand the principles of pretreatment.
2. Patient education can be pivotal in the success of the treatment and final outcome.
3. Patient selection has everything to do with an optimal outcome.
4. Patient selection refers to the physical, emotional, and intellectual candidacy.
5. Technology can be challenging and not always the right choice for the patient.
6. Just because it is new does not mean it is better.
7. Every procedure has risk. Understand and communicate these risks to your patient.
8. Close follow-up care and communication will sustain the patient-caregiver relationship.
9. Optimal outcomes to each procedure are in the hands of the clinician and the patient.
10. The clinician has to know his or her "stuff" to achieve an optimal outcome.

CHAPTER REVIEW QUESTIONS

1. Why is patient education important to ensure an optimal outcome?
2. What are the common aesthetic procedures used to improve appearance?
3. Why is patient selection important to an optimal outcome?
4. How can indications and contraindications overlap causing a challenge for the optimal outcome?
5. What has reality TV taught us about our appearance-obsessed society?

BIBLIOGRAPHY

Aesthetic. (2005, May 27). *ClearLight™ and Clear100™*. [Online]. Available: http://www.aesthetic.lumenis.com

Syneron Medical Aesthetics Technology. (2005, May 27). [Online]. Available: http://www.syneron.com

Thermage. (2005, May 27). [Online]. Available: http://www.thermage.com

Tsao, A. (2004, November 30). The changing face of skin care. *Business Week On-Line*. [Online]. Available: www.yahoo.businessweek.com

Tsao, A. (2004, November 30). Despite the hype, no elixirs of youth. *Business Week On-Line*. [Online]. Available: www.yahoo.businessweek.com

Glossary

A

active listening The process by which the receiver of information is paying attention to verbal and nonverbal cues as a means to understand fully the message the sender intends.

adaptation An adjustment to cultural surroundings.

B

body dysmorphic disorder A psychosocial disorder that causes individuals to be inappropriately concerned with their appearance. Persons affected with BDD are contraindicated for most aesthetic procedures.

Botox® Trade name for small doses of the botulism toxin (*Clostridium botulinum*) that are injected into the wrinkle-causing muscles. The toxin blocks the release of the chemicals that would otherwise signal the muscle to contract, thus paralyzing the injected muscle

bottom-up listening strategy A listening strategy during which the receiver uses grammar and word choice to understand the intended message of the sender.

C

character The features or traits of an individual.

collagen An insoluble protein found in connective tissues. Particularly, type I collagen forms a network in the epidermis, and it is credited with providing skin with its tensile strength and firmness.

communication The transmission of information by use of symbols.

complications Unexpected events that occur following a normally applied procedure.

conflict resolution The act of creating solutions to problems.

consequentialist ethics Psychologic traits; the outcome of the situation is most important.

consultation The initial visit with a professional during which the client and the professional both investigate whether a specific treatment or service is warranted or achievable.

contraindications Any sign or symptom indicating that a particular treatment, which would otherwise be advisable, would be inappropriate.

Cosmoderm® and Cosmoplast® Dermal fillers that are a variation on traditional bovine collagen using human collagen.

D

dermabrasion Predecessor to microdermabrasion that used a wire brush or a diamond-coated wheel to resurface the skin from the papillary dermal level.

dynamic rhytids   Wrinkling that occurs as a result of facial movement.

dyschromias   Skin discoloration.

E

ego   The "I" of someone.

empathy   Using thoughts, words, and actions as a means of conveying a deep level of understanding.

encoding   Part of communication that deals with translating ideas into symbols, such as words or letters, to best enable the receiver's understanding.

ethics   Moral values or principles.

external noises   Any outside distractions that interfere with the comprehension of a sender's message.

extrinsic aging   Changes that are brought on by the effects of the environment and our choices relating to them, specifically sunlight exposure.

F

fad   A temporary fashion or manner of conduct.

fictional finalism   The perfect self as described by Adler.

Fitzpatrick skin typing worksheet   A method of skin typing that considers the patient's complexion, hair color, eye color, ethnicity, and reaction to unprotected sunlight exposure.

functional needs   The needs that cause a society to exist.

G

glabella   The area of skin between the eyebrows, the underlying muscle groups of which cause creasing, or "frown lines," as a result of repeated squinting or frowning over time.

glycosaminoglycans   Polysaccharide chains, most prominent in the dermis, that bind with water, smoothing and softening the surface from below.

granulomas   A tumor caused by foreign bodies.

goal attainment   A term used to define objectives.

ground substance   A substance that consists mainly of glycosaminoglycans (hyaluronic acid, chondroitin sulfate, and dermatan sulfate) involved in maintenance and repair of dermis.

H

health history sheet   A document used by medical professionals to gather information on past and present health conditions, as well as the likelihood for future conditions. This sheet includes allergies, medical conditions, and prescription information.

Help Us Understand You sheet   A document that should be used by skin-care professionals to gauge a client's knowledge, expectations, and concerns so that the treatment will be mutually advantageous. This information is also used to differentiate the business and identify with the client.

human condition   The situation of being human.

Hylaform®   A dermal filler using animal-based hyaluronic acid.

I

id   The unconscious psyche; seeking pleasure.

idea   The beginning step of communication. Concepts and thoughts are translated into symbols and sent to the intended receiver.

image business   A type of business on which the way the public views the company is based largely on how things look, or how they are perceived, more so than actual performance.

impressions   A collection of lasting opinions or judgments of something.

indications   Any sign or circumstance indicating that a particular treatment is appropriate or warranted.

individual   A single human being.

individual needs   Single human's necessities.

inferiority   Less than.

integration   The act of bringing together.

internal noises   Any distractions from within, such as wondering or closed mind, that inhibit the understanding of a sent message.

interpersonal communication   Also called dyadic communication, involves communication between one person to another.

intrinsic aging   Changes that would occur over time without the effects of any environmental factors.

L

latencies   A stage of development, present but not visible.

listening   An active process of understanding what a sender is meaning, even if the person does not verbally say so. Listening involves the translation of verbal and nonverbal cues to extrapolate a meaning.

listening strategies   The use of different types of listening to keep your focus while extracting the information you are intended to garner.

M

magnetic resonance imaging   A noninvasive diagnostic technique that produces computerized images of internal body tissues.

metacognitive listening strategy   Using of both top-down and bottom-up strategies simultaneously to garner the messages most effectively. Persons who use this strategy will be best served in a particular situation: they monitor their comprehension and switch to another strategy if they believe their comprehension goals are not being met.

N

necrosis   The death of cells when tissue is deprived of blood supply.

nonsurgical aesthetic skin care   Any noninvasive procedure that is intended to improve overall skin health and appearance.

nonverbal communication   A type of interpersonal communication whereby the sending of a message is accomplished without a verbal cue. This task is usually accomplished with hand signals, gesturing, posturing, and eye movements.

P

paradigm   A model or pattern.

patient information sheet   A document used by medical professionals to gather social, personal, and demographic information.

perception   Cognitive awareness or recognition. What the patient thinks of you.

personal ethics   Personal values.

phenol   A highly corrosive acid used in peel solutions, which dissolves cells to make room for newer and healthier ones.

prejudice   An unfavorable opinion.

principled ethics   Morals or principles that everyone should know and understand.

professional code of ethics   The morals held in common by a group of professionals.

professional ethics   Guidelines of behavior for the professional.

Propionibacterium acnes   Produces acne

psychology   The science of the mind.

R

radio frequency A frequency of transmitting radio waves.

regulations An authoritative rule dealing with details or procedure.

Restylane® A dermal filler using non-animal—based hyaluronic acid.

S

self-aware The ability to assess the situation without the emotional attachment.

side effects An action or effect of a drug other than that desired, such as nausea or vomiting.

skin history sheet A document used by skin-care professionals to gather information on a client's past and present skin health. This sheet includes past treatment, sunburns, and conditions that are necessary for treatment.

social atomism Organizational elements.

society An organized group of persons; religious, scientific, political, or otherwise.

sociology The study of human organizations.

static rhytids Wrinkling that occurs without reference to facial movement.

superego The conscience, formed early in life at the direction of parents and other behavioral role models.

T

telangiectasia Small visible capillaries sometimes referred to as broken capillaries.

Thermage® A noninvasion radio-frequency technology to improve facial appearance.

top-down listening strategy The listener uses background knowledge on the subject or the person for the purpose of listening for main ideas, predicting, drawing conclusions, and summarizing.

treatment consequences Predictable outcomes of the procedure that occur in a reasonable percentage of people having the procedure.

treatment history A period that is long enough to assess results, usually 2 years.

treatment plan A plan of action for patient care.

trends A prevailing tendency.

trichloroacetic acid A chemical used in peel solutions that dissolve aging cells to make room for newer, healthier ones.

V

verbal communication Type of interpersonal communication that involves the use of symbols, particularly words and other sounds, to send information to a recipient.

virtue ethics The principles of character.

Index